AN UNCERTAIN JOURNEY

One Couple Navigating a Health Crisis Through Uncharted Territory

KATHRYN LEIGH CRAWFORD
&
DAVID KENNEDY MCCULLOCH

BLUE FORGE PRESS
Port Orchard ✱ Washington

An Uncertain Journey

First eBook Edition, January 2020
First Print Edition, January 2020
Second Print Edition February 2023

ISBN 978-1-59092-839-4

Blue Forge Press is the print division of the volunteer-run, federal 501(c)3 nonprofit company, Blue Forge Group, founded in 1989 and dedicated to bringing light to the shadows and voice to the silence. We strive to empower storytellers across all walks of life with our four divisions: Blue Forge Press, Blue Forge Films, Blue Forge Gaming, and Blue Forge Records. Find out more at www.BlueForgeGroup.org

Blue Forge Press
7419 Ebbert Drive Southeast
Port Orchard, Washington 98367
blueforgepress@gmail.com
360-550-2071 ph.txt

"Be kind, for everyone you meet is fighting a hard battle."

—Plato

AN UNCERTAIN JOURNEY

One Couple Navigating a Health Crisis Through Uncharted Territory

KATHRYN LEIGH CRAWFORD

&

DAVID KENNEDY McCULLOCH

INTRODUCTION

Dave

The narrative in these pages was never written with the intention of it becoming a book. It was written during a tumultuous period in our lives when Kathryn and I had to deal with a life threatening illness requiring a prolonged, complicated, and dangerous treatment course. It is a series of journal entries, each written in the moment as we both faced rapidly changing new realities. The primary purpose of these journal entries was to give day-to-day updates to our close friends and family so that Kathryn and I would not have to keep repeating the same answers to the same questions repeatedly. We used a website called Caring Bridge which makes it easy to share updates and support for a healing community.

As I started writing these updates it became clear to me that they were fulfilling two additional functions for me. I had thought I might write a separate private journal throughout the evolving treatment to document how it was affecting me but the physical and emotional demands of the illness and our response to it left me with so little extra energy that these Caring Bridge entries became my personal journal. They are written with raw emotion of how each of us was feeling at that moment, as we had to adjust to new and evolving circumstances. I am a writer and it helps me to process and cope better if I can write things down and explain things clearly to myself. Some of the journal entries give medical details that may be of interest only to our medical friends. Other entries are personal reflections to help me put things in perspective. Finally, these journal entries have allowed me to express how I feel about my remarkable partner, Kathryn Crawford.

First let me give a little bit of background about each of us. I grew up in a remote, rural part of Scotland where my father was the headmaster of a tiny two-person school in a hamlet called Mahaar. I went to high school in the seaside town of Ayr, went from there to Medical School in Edinburgh at age 17, and have pursued a career in medicine ever since. I moved to Seattle in 1983 so have now spent about half of my life in Scotland and the other half in the Pacific Northwest of the USA.

At the time this journal starts Kathryn and I had just turned sixty, and were living in Seattle in the Magnolia neighborhood very near to Discovery Park. We had five grown kids, three of whom were married with kids of their own, and though we are close to all of them emotionally they were living far apart across the USA.

We both feel incredibly fortunate. By the cosmic luck of where we popped up on the planet, the color of our skin, the opportunities we have had, and the careers we have been able to pursue, we were in a good position emotionally, financially, and geographically to deal with this adversity. We also had good health insurance. In 2014 there wasn't a better place on the planet to undergo the treatment that Kathryn chose than Seattle.

Growing up in Scotland in the 1950's I never dreamed that I would end up living in the USA. I have weathered critical looks from liberal Seattleites when I state, without apology, that I have five children. Don't I know that there are too many humans on the planet already and that they are causing climate change?! Humans should stop having children to save the planet. I don't mean to belittle those concerns or to minimize this very real problem. There are a lot of people on the planet. But I would argue that there are not too many *good* people on the planet. I believe that our children and grandchildren will be forces for good in the future of the world. And I know for certain that the world is a better place because Kathryn Crawford in still in it.

Kathryn will give her own introduction, but I'd like to say a few things about her. She has been reluctant about publishing our story. She is a modest and private person and felt that so many other people in the world have been through much more suffering or have much more exciting and interesting stories to tell than we do. I agree that there are tons of incredibly important stories to tell out there and I hope that many will be told. But I feel that many people will be able to relate to our story and may find it relevant to their own lives.

Kathryn

Dave is right. I have been reluctant to publish our Caring Bridge entries, in part because there are many more compelling stories out there. I am also not sure it will be useful in any way to others. Our kids might like a copy of this for posterity. They did read Caring Bridge but we had a separate family network of communication at the same time we were writing Caring Bridge. I do imagine that many people can relate to a story that is simply about a regular couple who had some bad luck on the health front. Although we all know now that our lifestyles affect our health, living a healthy lifestyle comes with no *guarantees* of good health. We should all do the best we can but, as a nurse, I feel like it's unfortunate that it's now to the point that people with health problems are sometimes blamed for them. For me, the purpose of the Caring Bridge writing was useful for two reasons. It was an efficient way for us to let family and friends know what was going on. In addition, it meant that the limited time I had to spend with people could be spent talking about the world, or about *them*, not my body. I did not find my interest in other people waning during my treatment. I guess one purpose of publishing might be that people who are grappling with serious health issues might feel fortified knowing they have company out there as they forge on through difficult circumstances and uncertainty.

In my situation the two treatment options were stark. One was to accept worsening symptoms and die slowly in a year or two. The alternative was to receive a stem cell transplant, *if* a donor could be found, and potentially be cured of myelofibrosis. However, with a transplant there were no guarantees that I would survive the treatment, live and wish I hadn't, or do fairly well and have an acceptable quality of life. I have often described the treatment as being both barbaric and miraculous. I would be hospitalized and have my immune system blasted out with toxic drugs—the barbaric part. The drugs are very blunt instruments and they damage healthy body parts as well as the cancerous immune system. Meanwhile the donor cells would be retrieved from the donor and flown back to the Seattle Cancer Care Alliance and infused into me within thirty-six hours. If I was lucky, the cells would figure out where to go and what they were supposed to do. They were supposed to find their way into my bone marrow and begin making healthy blood. That's the miraculous part.

Even though I would die without a transplant, I gave serious consideration to each option. I wrote out a fairly detailed "thought experiment" outlining how each option might go and sent it to a few friends for discussion. This is a decision point in many serious illnesses when the sick person often feels a lot of pressure from friends or family to get the most intensive treatment, even if it may not help much. Some people actually live longer when they have a focus on their present quality of life with the help of hospice services. Sometimes getting straight answers about how likely a treatment is to be effective requires being very assertive. It helps a lot if there are frank conversations about treatment pros and cons, and clarification about whose decision it really is. In my case, the treatment would be brutal but there was definitely some realistic hope of survival imbedded in getting the transplant that wasn't there if I decided against it. I worked toward a state of equanimity about living or dying. I was worried about how either one would affect Dave and my family. Dave and I talked a lot about how either path would affect our relationship, what the biggest stressors would probably be, and how he would get support if I couldn't give him much. We have wonderful kids but they live out of state and we felt strongly that they needed to get on with their lives. Without me, I knew Dave could have a healthy partner and do all the things he and I had imagined we would do in our sixties. I took care of my mother, who had dementia, for ten years and she had died just before my diagnosis. Dave and I then had big plans since our children were launched and my mom was gone. I knew our kids would miss me if I died but I also knew they would be fine. We have been conscious of wanting to help frame this whole experience in a way that may help our adult children recognize that we can all learn and grow in unique ways from suffering, it isn't all bad.

I experienced what I have referred to as a "hope conundrum." On the one hand, I was told that the people who are most satisfied with post-transplant life were those who were very worried about dying and who had low expectations. On the other, we are all told that we should go into any major medical treatment with great optimism and determination that we are going to "beat this thing." There is some tension between the two ways of thinking about the treatment. I'm a bit surprised that I have never gone back and read our Caring Bridge entries until Dave expressed an interest in publishing them. My main three hopes were that if I survived the transplant I would be able to think and read and be physically active.

The issue of "fairness" came up often. Many people suggested that it wasn't fair that I should have something so lethal after exercising, eating my vegetables, and keeping my stress level in check for my entire adult life. The comment felt alienating to me since I didn't feel that way at all. I figured out by the time I was twenty that life wasn't fair, and recognized that I had gotten way more than my share of the good stuff in life. The comment that I found most reassuring throughout the whole ordeal was that I just seemed like myself.

Luckily for me, I am usually able to find difficulty interesting and I am also grateful for a multitude of things. I managed to hang onto my sense of humor even though I did notice that more of my humor was black. I went through all of this with wonderful support from family and friends, expert and caring providers, good insurance, enough money, and a wonderful place to live. Besides all that, I have a partner who is smart, industrious, good humored, and a person of great depth. He managed my complicated home regimen of medications, dressing changes, and IV infusions, he cooked and did laundry, and he drove me to all my appointments. He was prepared to be by my side every step of the way. And that made all the difference.

SETTING THE STAGE

This was the letter that Dave sent to all of our kids when we first found out about the diagnosis and what was being proposed:

Sunday, March 2nd 2014

Life, itself, is an uncertain journey, of course but when you or someone you love is diagnosed with something bad the uncertainty of life is brought into stark relief. We have known since 2005 that Kathryn has Polycythemia Vera, a (hopefully) slow growing cancer of the cells that make blood in the bone marrow. Our recent news suggests that the nature of this is changing in ways that are not good but just how bad the news is we won't know for a few more weeks. It is clear that there will be many ups and downs during this adventure. I would like to suggest a few "ground rules" that we should think about that might make this easier (and richer) for all of us. This is an incomplete list, and you can feel free to add more or modify these as you see fit, but here are some things that occur to me today that may be helpful to each of us in different ways.

Ground Rules for the Uncertain Journey

Communication. Share what you want with whomever you want and respect each other's privacy. This journey affects all of us in different ways. We all have different coping strategies and will want to give and receive support in different ways. We are all close, honest, and authentic with each other. There are some things that Kathryn or I will want to share with everyone, but we do not expect responses to always be to the whole group. There are things you may want to ask Kathryn by herself, or there may be things you want to share with just me, or with each other.

Compartmentalize. Kathryn and I do not want to turn into gloomy walking medical textbooks dwelling constantly on the minutiae of research on myeloproliferative neoplasms. Rest assured that we will take on the medical system at Seattle Cancer Care Alliance and elsewhere with gusto, intelligence and determination and will leave no stone unturned to figure out the best path for Kathryn's future quality and quantity of life. But we all need to remember that "regular life" has to go on for us and for everyone else, too. We need to try to compartmentalize areas of our life so that we find time to rejoice in other things.

Humor. Let's continue to share humor (including gallows humor!) as we come across it. It helps both Kathryn and me a lot to find things to laugh about through all of this.

Feelings. At various times any of us may feel anger, sadness, impatience, frustration or any number of other emotions. Feel free to share any of these with Kathryn, me, or each other.

Individual hopes and dreams. Just because Kathryn's health will become a bigger part of what she and I need to think about on a day-to-day basis it does not mean that we care any less about what is going on in all of your lives. We love you all dearly and are intensely interested in the day-to-day goings on and the short and long term plans that you all have. Communication between us should NOT always be about Kathryn's health. We want to continue to hear about your current worries, frustrations, joys and successes and what your hopes and plans are for the short and long term future.

Living in the now. I am not very knowledgeable about Buddhism or meditation or other disciplines that emphasize training oneself to become better tuned in to appreciating and contemplating the here and now of everyday life. I do, though, try to do that in my own way. Feel free to share any wisdom that any of you have about that.

Spirituality. We are all different in how we imagine our place in the universe, the "purpose" of our lives, and what has come before or may come afterwards. I was raised in a very complacent middle-class tradition of Scottish Presbyterianism that was about as unspiritual, unhelpful, and un-meaningful as it could be in guiding how I lived my life. I won't launch into a diatribe about how little I think of "organized religion" of all stripes (although I will be happy to expand on that to any of you who want to discuss this). We all have every right to imagine anything we like about the unknowns about our current or future existence. I just hope that none of us will try to proselytize to each other about any of this. I certainly don't want to hear platitudes about "God working in mysterious ways" through all of this and I don't think Kathryn does either (ask her, though, if you want to know her thoughts).

Share. Jokes, poems, encouragement, Corgi videos on YouTube, or anything else that you think some others may enjoy, too.

Thanks for your love and support and for staying in touch whenever you can.

PATIENCE AND PREPARATION

Dave

Mar 22, 2014

This is my first entry on Caring Bridge. I will plan to post entries on a fairly regular basis but have no expectation that people need to respond to them. I will post a mixture of things, some practical, some amusing, others more reflective. At this point both Kathryn and I are just waiting and preparing the best we can for what is coming up. I ordered a dense little pocket manual that is used by Hematopoetic Stem Cell Transplant (HSCT) Team members and am immersing myself in a lot of complex and terrifying details about all the drugs, potential side effects, complications that can arise, and what can be done for each of them. It feels overwhelming and the idea that we will have to face all of these issues is daunting. However, I am reminded (and try to remind

Kathryn who will have to deal with these more intensely than the rest of us) that they may not all happen and that they won't happen all at once.

It really does feel like it is best to take things in phases and to just keep pacing ourselves. During this "Pre-HSCT" phase I am trying to learn about what things I will need to be particularly careful about when KC comes home from the hospital to rest and recover. Infection prevention and food handling safety are **very** high on the list of things to concentrate on. So you can look forward to getting riveting posts about those details in due course! You can skip those posts, of course if you find they are putting you off your own food...

We are trying to retain our sense of humor, stay patient, and get prepared.

AN UNEASY CALM BEFORE THE...?

Dave

June 7, 2014

It's not like me to be stuck for words, but I hesitate to use the word "storm" in this situation. Metaphors about storms, wars, or battles are often used for people dealing with cancer but for Kathryn and me those don't feel quite right. Yes, there will be times when we feel like we are fighting angrily and defiantly against an unkind and unforgiving foe, but given how long this struggle is going to go on I want to use a more positive and optimistic metaphor. I'll return to that later...

The past three months have tested our patience. We both feel nervous about what lies ahead. We have devoured textbooks, websites, and review papers and now know about every possible problem and side effect that might occur. We also realize that the alternatives of "doing nothing," or "letting nature take its course" are even less appealing. We have reached the point where we just want to shrug, sigh, and say, "Let's get started." Except that we can't... not just yet.

About three weeks ago Kathryn got word from Laurie, her search coordinator that, because Kathryn has a very unusual combination of HLA genetic markers, the best they can find is a donor who is an imperfect 9 out of 10 match. In other words this person is identical to Kathryn in four of the five important pairs of HLA markers but in only one antigen in the last pair. Our wise and experienced oncologist at the Seattle Cancer Care Alliance met with us and said he thought that while this was not ideal it was still a very acceptable donor and that we should proceed. He also said that he wanted to present Kathryn's details to his colleagues at SCCA to get their collective wisdom, input, and suggestions about what would be the best way to proceed. I'll write more about that in a separate journal entry. It meant that we had to be patient for several more weeks.

We have two main tasks during this waiting period. We need to prepare ourselves as best we can, physically, mentally, and emotionally for what is to come, and prepare our home to be a great place to heal and recover. We have tackled all of this with typical McCulloch-Crawfordian gusto. We have been trying to fatten Kathryn up by 10-15 pounds since many patients lose that amount during the first 100 days and the "normal sized Kathryn" doesn't have fifteen pounds to spare! So we have been eating delicious food, in bigger portions, and having more dessert. Not an unpleasant task, I grant you, but I need to keep reminding myself that it is **Kath**, and not **me**, who is supposed to gain the weight!

At the end of every day in the early evening we drive to Discovery Park to walk the three-mile Loop Trail at a vigorous clip. This does us both good physically and mentally, allows us to gauge Kathryn's strength and stamina, and gives us a chance to check in on what is going on in the wider world, with our kids and grandkids, and with how we are both feeling. After dinner we have been "escaping" to Downton Abbey for an hour - a delightful distraction.

Preparing our home to be a healing place has meant sprucing up the garden to be even more colorful and charming than it usually is. We repainted the entryway and all the upstairs rooms to look and feel fresh and clean and cheerful. I threw out lots of old bookcases and dressers and have bought several new fresh pieces of pine furniture from IKEA for both the Magnolia house and our Vashon cabin. We wanted the cabin to be another cheerful, functional, restorative place where any of the kids and grandkids could go to get away from the stress of all of this for a bit.

So I have been doing a heavy dose of "some assembly required" tasks, staring at smiling Swedish cartoon characters demonstrating how to tell right-handed and left-handed wood panels apart, which dowels, screws, and bolts go where, and how to hold heavy pieces of wood in place without having five arms, eyes in the back of your head, suction cups on your finger tips, a spirit level on your forehead and the balance and poise of a professional ballerina. IKEA construction is, for me, a long, painful, achy, confusing process. I learned how to curse (in Scottish rather than Swedish) while holding a screwdriver between my teeth, learned how to stop the bleeding when I brought shelving crashing down on my head, and learned how to shrug and sigh when the finished product was imperfect. Some of the drawers might stick a little, some of the legs are a bit shoogly, a few of the shelves are out of alignment, and none of it could be described as being beautiful. But it all looks fresh, new, functional, and not unattractive.

And then it came to me! The perfect metaphor for what lies ahead. Helping Kathryn through all of this will be, for me, like taking on a really big, complicated IKEA project. The instructions will be complex and confusing. I will sometimes mess things up. The end product may be a little shaky, at first, may not be as beautiful as we might have hoped for, but we will end up with something that is really quite attractive, functional, and full of fresh possibilities for the future. Now **that's** a metaphor that I can get behind! Let's get started.

SO HERE'S THE PLAN...

Dave

June 7, 2014

The Seattle Cancer Care Alliance has been doing bone marrow (or now mostly stem cell) transplants for over four decades. When I was a young doctor-in-training in Edinburgh in the 1970s one of our young rising stars in the field of blood cancers took a two year fellowship at the Fred Hutch Cancer Research Center (now part of SCCA) to learn all the latest techniques. He came back evangelized to develop more "aggressive" and curative approaches to blood cancers. Much progress has been made since then and so protocols are constantly being modified to incorporate new ideas, new drugs, and new discoveries.

Like many people with the type of bone marrow cancer that Kathryn has, the cancer cells make a specific protein called JAK-2. Drugs are being developed to target JAK-2 in the hopes of slowing down or stopping the cancer. Those that have been developed so far (including one called ruxolitinib or "*Jakafi*") can slow things down a bit and may improve symptoms but have not been shown to prolong the person's life to any significant extent. They are mostly used to relieve symptoms in people who are too unwell to get a stem cell transplant. However, the latest thinking is that if someone like Kathryn gets treated with Jakafi for 6-8 weeks **before** getting high dose chemotherapy followed by the stem cell transplant the tumor might be rendered even more susceptible to that treatment and so it might increase the chance of a long term "cure." Probably won't hurt. Might help. So we are doing that. Kathryn is into her third week on Jakafi without too many side effects.

Things will start to ramp up for Kathryn starting on July 1st. Because so many people fly from all over the USA and elsewhere in the world to get cancer treatment at SCCA they have organized things to be done efficiently once the person arrives in Seattle. So even though we live just twenty minutes from SCCA Kathryn's "Arrival Date" will be July 1st. During the following two weeks she will have lots of appointments to talk to nurses, doctors, psychologists, nutritionists, and others. She will get poked and prodded, have blood tests, ECGs, bone marrow tests, lung function studies, and bone density tests among other things. She and I will then be summoned to a meeting with Kathryn's transplant team where a doctor will summarize the results of all these tests and explain what will happen next. If they think that Kathryn is physically fit enough to withstand it she will be admitted to the UW transplant unit where she will receive full "myeloablative conditioning." This consists of high dose chemotherapy for a week to destroy her bone marrow (and hopefully the tumor). Her hair will fall out and she will feel sick, nauseated, sleepy and weak. During this same week in a distant city, the young woman who is to be Kathryn stem cell donor will be receiving daily injections of colony-stimulating growth factor to rev up her healthy bone marrow to produce lots of "feisty," activated stem cells that will spill out into her blood. She will then be admitted to a local hospital for four hours so that they can skim off those stem cells from her blood, package them up in a solution to keep them "happy" and fly them back to Seattle to be infused into Kathryn's blood within 24 hours or so.

Kathryn will then stay in hospital for another 2-3 weeks while the new stem cells hopefully decide that they like their new neighborhood and will set up their new home in Kathryn's now "empty" bone marrow. Once they have settled in, chosen their color scheme, and picked out the furniture they like, they will hopefully start making healthy new red cells, white cells, and platelets.

If all goes well Kathryn would then be ready to be discharged home where I will continue to track what pills she needs, keep her central IV line clean and clear, give her safe, nutritious food, check her temperature, keep a look out for new symptoms or problems, and try to keep her as comfortable, cheerful, and happy as possible. I will take 4-6 weeks off work at that time to give Kathryn my full attention. If things go well, I should be able to get back to work, perhaps on a somewhat lighter schedule, initially. Cameron will be able to share the caregiver responsibilities with me at that point.

So that's the tentative plan. At every stage we need to be flexible about changes to that plan depending on how Kathryn responds. It is scary big stuff to deal with but for both Kathryn and me it feels good to **have** a plan and to be actively doing things that will help guide her to a better place in the future.

SOME ENCOURAGEMENT ON THE SUMMER SOLSTICE

Dave

June 22, 2014

Yesterday was a glorious sunny day in Seattle. But while many of the city residents were wandering through the Fremont Fair drinking in the beer garden and watching the now traditional naked cyclist parade Kathryn and I spent the day inside an auditorium at SCCA participating in the 5th Biennial conference on Marrow Failure sponsored by the Aplastic Anemia & MDS International Foundation. Now WE know how to have a good time!

While not all of the lectures (from experts at SCCA, Mayo clinic, Cleveland Clinic and elsewhere) were directly relevant to what Kathryn has it gave us a great sense of the rapid rate of progress in understanding how to manage and treat these kinds of diseases to increase the rate of "cure" and improve the quality of life. I came away with two big takeaways, one of a scientific nature and the other about the importance of what pyscho-social things we can do to have a healthy perspective on how life might be different after transplant.

The big "Ah-Ha" that I got on the scientific front is that the drug that Kathryn has been started on, ruxolitinib (Jakafi) is just the first or second in a line of promising new therapies. It has been shown to improve symptoms a lot, in some people shrink the spleen, and even prolong life by about a year in people who are not suitable for a stem cell transplant. All that is encouraging. Certainly Kathryn has found that it has given her more energy and has made fairly dramatic changes to her weekly blood counts such that her dose has had to be adjusted twice already. The most encouraging thing was to hear Dr. Deeg say that he and other experts in the field think that by pre-treating someone like Kathryn with ruxolitinib for 6-8 weeks it will reduce the inflammation in her bone marrow and change and weaken the tumor so that there should be three benefits. **First**, it will speed up the time to engraftment. That means that when the donor stem cells are infused they will find the environment within the bone marrow less hostile and so will take up residence faster. Kathryn will be most vulnerable to life-threatening infections and bleeding during the days after her own bone marrow has been destroyed until the new stem cells start making red cells, white cells and platelets so if pretreatment with ruxolitinib will make that happen faster so much the better. **Second**, with the tumor weakened by ruxolitinib the new stem cells will be able to destroy the remaining tumor cells more effectively and so the likelihood of Kathryn's myelofibrosis coming back will be reduced.

And **third**, They believe that pretreatment with ruxolitinib will make conditions enough better for the incoming stem cells that they will be "happier" in their new home and so the risk of chronic graft-versus-host-disease (GVHD) will be reduced. Let's hope that all three of these things come to pass.

Ruben Mesa, MD, from the Mayo Clinic in Arizona, gave a very thoughtful talk about how to think about "surviving" stem cell transplantation. We shouldn't think about it as being hellish for some set amount of time and then at some mythical date in the future Kathryn will be "cured" and be off all drugs with the same quality of life that she had before she was ever diagnosed. We will always have to live with some uncertainty (about myelofibrosis coming back or GVHD rearing its ugly head, or indeed like everyone else of our age, that some other unrelated illness will strike one of us). Rather we should live in ways to maximize our enjoyment and energy for ourselves and to give to others. He gave his top ten countdown list of things to do to maximize our future quality of life. Now while most of the things on this list are common sense and should apply to all of us whether or not we are facing an illness like Kathryn's, I still thought it was a list worth sharing with you.

10. Learn about the disease - but not TOO much! This one certainly resonates with both of us. We have dived into the literature on myeloproliferative neoplasms with vigor and have learned a ton so that we understand what is being done and why. But knowing about every POSSIBLE side effect and thing that could go wrong can get a person feeling pessimistic so we are tempering our academic enthusiasm for knowledge with a certain amount of willful ignorance. We don't need to know

EVERYTHING.

9. **Make friends with others facing similar challenges.** Kathryn has done a great job of this and has reached out to several other individuals who have had stem cell transplants for a variety of reasons. She has listened to how they coped at the various stages, learned what their support structure was like and what things they think they did well and what they might have done differently. While no one person's journey is the same as another person's it is helpful to get some perspective.

8. **Be your own best advocate.** Dealing with this disease is complicated stuff with drugs, visits, lab tests and e-mails between many different people in different organizations (Group Health, SCCA, UWMC) who don't necessarily talk to each other so we need to be assertive enough to make sure that communication is as good as it can be and that WE know what is going on. Luckily neither of us is a shrinking violet...

7. **Capture what is discussed at doctor's visits by having a friend there or recording what was said to listen to later.** This is smart advice. To this point we have not recorded the visits that we have had with Dr. Deeg but we did find that comparing notes with each other afterwards has been very helpful. We sometimes hear things differently or interpret what was said differently. During the first two weeks in July when Kathryn and I will be going to several big meetings where several people in our transplant team will be telling us LOTS of things we may well ask their permission to record the visit on one of our iPhones.

6. **Take care of your caregiver.** I especially liked this piece of advice! (Although in truth he needs to take care of himself to make sure he is in his best form to help

Kathryn get through all of this).

5. Take care of the rest of your health. Again, this is common sense and something that we should all try to do all of the time.

4. Eat in a healthy way (at least most of the time ;-). This comes easily to us and we both understand that having the occasional slice of homemade lemon meringue pie **IS** healthy for the body... and soul.

3. Exercise, exercise, exercise. He couldn't emphasize enough that when you are feeling weak and exhausted it is easy to give yourself a "pass" and just sit still or lie down. Just like astronauts in space and athletes who get laid up with a broken leg it is amazing how quickly your muscles atrophy and so you feel even weaker and give yourself another pass and so get even weaker. I have never known anyone as determined and dedicated to regular exercise as Kathryn Crawford is but I know it is going to be hard for her in the first 100 days after the stem cell transplant. She and I are talking about strategies to help her keep doing some amount of exercise every day if at all possible. Since she will be confined to the house for much of that time and since public gymnasia and sports clubs are cesspools of bacteria, fungi, and viruses we plan to set up a compact, Standing "Total Gym" in her office upstairs next to the treadmill. I can use this, too, to try to keep the caregiver healthy.

2. Live every moment to the fullest. Great advice for anyone, of course. The point he was making in the setting of an illness like Kathryn's is that you should try not to just grin-and-bear-it dourly in the hope that there will be some mythical day in the future when you will "feel better." We will certainly try to find something to laugh about every day, focus on how others are doing, appreciate small pleasures, and stay optimistic.

1. Focus on relationships. We really both do that anyway. This is the most rewarding and valuable and treasured part of our existence, always has been and always will be.

So we ended yesterday by going for a brisk walk round Discovery Park (3), talking about the information we got at the conference (10), discussed the other people we had met at the conference (9), compared notes (7), enjoyed the exquisite smells and sounds of summer in the woods (2), made each other laugh (6), chatted about how all our kids and grandkids were doing (1), and came home to eat a delicious vegan pasta salad on the deck with Cameron (4, 5, 2, 1). A very good day overall.

DEPENDENCE DAY?

Dave

July 4, 2014

I love this country. Having lived almost half my life in the USA and having been a proud US citizen since 1988 I can say that July 4th means a lot to me. I love the brash optimism of our citizens, the simplistic ways in which we consider our relationship with the rest of the world. And yet as someone with dual citizenship, who grew up in sleepy, rural Scotland in the 1950s and 1960s, I also see the USA with an affectionate objectivity. I have spent many, many July 4ths with Kathryn's extended family at the beach on Vashon Island experiencing America's annual celebration of beer, sunburn, and explosives...

There have only been two times since 1987 when I have not been part of July 4th celebrations. The first was in 2002. Kath and I spent a glorious month in France with Cameron and Murray tootling around in our tiny Citroen car traveling from the blistering heat and lavender fields of the South of France, west to the lush valleys and limestone cave paintings of the Dordogne valley, north to the decadent, ostentatious castles of the Loire valley and back to the delightfully seedy Parisian neighborhood of Montmartre. July 4th, 2002, found us paddling down the Dordogne River on a calm sunny day. Cameron and Murray were baffled why no one was shooting off fireworks or grilling hot dogs... It was a great teaching moment for us about international perspectives on life. This concept was brought home even more starkly to the boys ten days later when we were living in our apartment in Paris on July 14th, "Quatorze Juillet," "Bastille Day," when drunken Parisians (along with busloads of tourists) shoot off fireworks and sing their lungs out into the humid night air above the city in celebration of **their** independence from tyrannical rule.

Today, July 4th, 2014, is the second time that I have not felt part of the typical American family's celebration of our country's independence. Both Kathryn and I are in the USA, for sure, in our home in Seattle, Washington. But we don't feel like being part of the usual extended family celebrations on Vashon this year. We saw many of those folk a few weeks ago when we held an open house to thank everyone for their support and to give everyone as much information as they felt comfortable with about what Kathryn has, and what she is facing. So today we don't want to be wet blankets and "downers" on everyone else's exuberant and lighthearted celebrations. There is really nothing very "light" about our lives right now. Three days of intense "arrival events" at SCCA (of which I will write more in a separate journal entry) has made us feel more "dependent" than we ever have in our lives before. I feel as though we are being sucked slowly but irreversibly into a very, very long tunnel and that neither of us knows how long that tunnel is, what shape we will be in when we emerge, or just how much "independence" we will feel in our lives from that point onwards. I hope that we will feel that we have a LOT of independence in the future, a lot of energy, fortitude, and an adventurous spirit. We may not be able to do everything we once thought might be possible but we will be flexible and creative in our outlook. Kathryn Crawford is one of the most independent thinkers and the most stubborn, curious and independent spirits I have ever known. I am confident that our future will certainly be interesting and full of adventures of one sort or another. It is a privilege and honor to share this day with her. Happy Fourth!

WHAT DAY IS THIS ANYWAY?

Dave

July 4, 2014

For Kathryn and me our lives are being broken up into (hopefully) manageable "bite sized" pieces that are tied to **days** and **dates**. Tuesday, July 1st, 2014, was Kathryn's "**Arrival Date**" in Seattle, as far as the Seattle Cancer Care Alliance (SCCA) was concerned. As someone who has lived around Seattle for most of her life and vividly remembers going to the World's Fair to see the Space Needle in 1962 this seems an odd concept. However, since 90% of SCCA patients travel from elsewhere around the country and the wider world to get their care here SCCA has refined its approach to be as efficient as possible. Between Kathryn's "arrival day" and the day she will get her stem cell transplant (**Day Zero!**) there is a lo-o-o-ot to be done.

We have met several members of our transplant team. We are on the **TAN Team** (as opposed to the Blue Team or the Orange Team). Being on the Tan Team seems a little ironic to me since they never cease to emphasize that Kathryn must **NOT** be exposed to the sun unless she is slathered in SPF-50 sunscreen spread half an inch thick and is wearing eighteen layers of long-sleeved clothing and a giant sombrero hat! Tan, she will not be...

Other days and dates are firmly locked into our consciousness, too. Kathryn started ruxolitinib (Jakafi) on May 16th, 2014, so today is **Day 50** of Jakafi. She needs to be tapered off this drug before she gets her conditioning chemotherapy (tentatively scheduled for July 18th, which would then be **Day -7**). Ruxolitinib cannot be stopped abruptly and so we start to taper it on the afternoon of July 7th (**Day -18**) and stop it altogether on the morning of July 17th (**Jakafi Day 63** or **Day -8** depending on how you look at it).

In order to keep all of this straight I have set up my "Caregiver's organization corner" near one of my infamous some-assembly-required-IKEA-dressers. On a bulletin board above the dresser I keep a copy of Kath's SCCA upcoming appointment schedule and have created a spreadsheet to keep track of the ever-changing drugs that she is taking and the varying doses of those drugs at different times and on different days. Since many of these need to be taken with food we now have a very different look on our bedside table these days. Pillboxes and magazines about headscarves didn't used to be regular items in our daily lives.

Day -7 is the day that Kathryn gets admitted to the University of Washington's Transplant Unit to start her conditioning chemotherapy. Since that will make her vulnerable to infections like Pneumocystis she has been started on the prophylactic antibiotic, Bactrim, (on **Day -21**). Since that might interact with her conditioning chemotherapy or with the stem cell transplant (I think) this is to be stopped on either **Day -9** or **Day -2** (we need to verify which one).

Day 0 is the date when the donor stem cells are infused into Kathryn's body. Our transplant nurse, Pat, a friendly, bustling, bright, experienced, and plain-spoken (which we appreciate) woman said to us, **Day 0** doesn't start until the stem cell infusion is completed. So if they start infusing them at 10pm on Friday July 25th but the infusion isn't completed until 2am on Saturday July 26th then July 26th is **Day 0**, and not July 25th. Don't you be thinking that you can slip an extra day in there to shorten the misery!

Everything important is tracked from **Day 0**. Kathryn will be most vulnerable to bleeding and infections in the first 20+ days so she will have daily blood tests, and will be given more prophylactic antibiotics, antivirals, and antifungals. They will hope to see signs of engraftment of the new stem cells (as seen by rising white cell or platelet counts) between **Day 10** and **Day 25**. Kathryn should be discharged to home care between **Days 20** to **Day 30**. If all goes well we will have a major conference with our transplant team on **Day 80**. The target is to be discharged by the transplant team back to "usual care" by **Day 100** (although truthfully we will have a very different and ever-changing concept of "usual" after all of this and we will be lucky if things truly feel normal at **Day 365** or by **Day 1,095**...

All of these dates are tentative and subject to

change. We have been assured (not reassured!) that this whole process never goes totally smoothly for anyone. We just don't know which particular hiccups will occur for Kathryn, how bad they will be, or how long they will last.

So here we are. Greetings from your trying-to-stay-optimistic-but-vigilant-and-flexible friends on **Day -21ish**. Onwards and upwards.

AFTER "ARRIVAL..."

Kathryn

July 15, 2014

After a grueling two weeks of extensive physical exams, Dave and I were delighted to have some time with our wonderful family doing some "normal" things--barbecuing, cold drinks on sunny days, walking the beach at Discovery Park. All 5 kids, partners, and 6 grandkids were in one place (rare) and not much beats the sound of children squealing with delight on the beach. We savored all of it.

Now we are onto a week of preparation for full blast treatment beginning with admission to UW Hospital this Friday, probably for about a month. I am having a central line placed in my chest tomorrow to allow them to take blood and give me infusions without poking my arms each time. I "passed" the physical tests, which means that the SCCA team believes my body will be able to withstand the high dose chemotherapy regimen. Although this increases my risk of treatment related toxicities, it maximizes the chances of the new cells working and minimizes my chances of relapse. My biggest risk in the coming months/years is graft-versus-host-disease (GVHD). It commonly affects the skin, eyes, and mouth and can damage internal organs. The treatment involves continued immune suppression. Hopefully that will run its course in 3-4 years. The immune suppression drugs serve a purpose but prednisone, specifically, can also damage muscles, bones, internal organs and the ability to sleep.

Dave is taking this on in his characteristic can-do way. He's already gone to classes, watched the videos, and stocked up on bleach and squirt bottles. I am lucky indeed to have a loving caregiver taking on this role with zest. He will take some time off work when I am discharged and when he begins to return to work Cameron will take over as backup caregiver. We will really be trying to make the most of each day even as I begin my first chemotherapy infusion on Friday. I am thinking of it as making friends with toxins. I will focus on them clearing out my bone marrow so that I am able to provide a warm welcome for my new cells the following week.

It's unsettling to prepare to pay this high a price with no guarantees and long term uncertainty about what the outcome might be. We appreciate the offers of support and expect to need some as we discover what this path really involves day-to-day. I have no idea at all how I will feel and whether visitors will sound like a good idea. From what I've been told, it sounds like it might feel like an accomplishment just to put my clothes on in the morning. Dave will write about that here if I can't. The love and support we receive from all of you help us keep our spirits up and find the stamina we need to carry on. We continue to welcome jokes, humor of all kinds, poems and short story suggestions.

With gratitude to all of you,
Kathryn

DEEP BREATHS ALL AROUND

Kathryn

July 17, 2014

Well, the day has finally come for my family and me to begin this long, uncertain journey. I now have my new chest rig that involves a flexible catheter placed near my heart. Two branches come out on my chest and allow the infusion of incompatible medications simultaneously. It will also be used for frequent blood draws. If I'm lucky, I will be rid of it in a few months but I may well have it for a year.

We have learned a lot about managing at home after the hospital and it won't be simple. The emphasis is on careful attention to avoiding infections. We have learned about how to do effective cleaning of our house and we really need to up our game in that department (!)

Dave is gearing up for delicious cooking that meets the requirements. My policy on rules is to know what they are and then decide whether or not to follow them. We plan to follow every one with care for the foreseeable future.

An unlikely request from me--For any of you who might think I'd like some flowers, you'd be right. However, I cannot have ANY flowers or plants in the hospital or house for the rest of the year. Luckily, we have a LOT of them in the front yard.

I feel like we are about as ready for this as we can be. We have really had time to think this decision through and prepare as best we can. We feel like we are in very good hands and that counts for a lot. We will take great comfort from each other and from your support. This will be a major exercise in taking each day as it comes, and having faith that we will have what it takes to stay calm and grounded amidst the ups and downs.

A poem that reminds me that what we need is here:

The Wild Geese

Horseback on Sunday morning,
harvest over, we taste persimmon
and wild grape, sharp sweet
of summer's end. In time's maze
over fall fields, we name names
that went west from here, names
that rest on graves. We open
a persimmon seed to find the tree
that stands in promise,
pale, in the seed's marrow.
Geese appear high over us,
pass, and the sky closes. Abandon,
as in love or sleep, holds
them to their way, clear,
in the ancient faith: what we need
is here. And we pray, not
for new earth or heaven, but to be
quiet in heart, and in eye
clear. What we need is here.

Love,
Kathryn

DAYS -7 AND -6

Dave

July 19, 2014

Yesterday was Kathryn's "Blast Off!" day (Day -7). Cameron and I got up early and came to the UWMC transplant unit with her to help her get settled in. Everyone on 7NE has been very pleasant, exuding competence and cheerfulness. Kathryn's nurse, Lynn, is slim, fiftyish, and originally from New York. She and Kathryn are getting along great. At this point things seem a bit anticlimactic. Kathryn still looks great and feels fine despite the continuous infusions of saline, dexamethasone, lorazapam, baclofen, ondansetron, and then an hour-long infusion of cyclophosphamide (Cytoxan). This is the first of the "big guns" that will flatten her own immune system so that she will accept the new stem cells that she will get next week. Kathryn didn't get any of the expected nausea or hiccups with the

Cytoxan and has been ordering and eating food with some gusto. I stayed with her all day while Cameron left to run some errands. He got back around 5pm so I left then to get back home to do house chores. Cameron and later Murray hung out with Kath during the evening after Murray was done with work (he is doing construction for the summer and has spent the past several days putting siding on a big new house in Ballard while learning new elaborate and creative combinations of cuss words from his co-workers).

This morning (Day -6) when I came in Kathryn was walking the triangular loop within the transplant unit doing her "laps" to keep her energy up and help get rid of the leg edema that builds up with the amount of intravenous saline she is getting to keep her kidneys well flushed. At this point she still has quite a spring in her step as she takes her constant companion (the IV pole on wheels to which is attached bags of fluids and a couple of infusion pumps) around and around the halls. She gets another large dose of Cytoxan today and then tomorrow starts the first of four days of busulfan. This second "big gun" of the conditioning regimen is the one that most directly and completely attacks the bone marrow to clean out both good and bad cells that are there. It is a drug that has been around for decades and many places give it orally and in a fixed dose. One of the things that SCCA/UWMC have pioneered is giving the busulfan intravenously and in a variable dose targeted to keep her blood level within a specific range to maximize the effectiveness of the drug while minimizing the side effects that it can have on her other organs.

As Kathryn and I walk the halls together we pass some of the other "inmates" who are plodding along with bald heads, and grim looks on their ashen gray faces. They will have a variety of different underlying diagnoses and are obviously a lot farther into the whole transplant process than Kathryn is but it is a stark reminder of what lies ahead for us. It is a dull gray day outside and we are both feeling a bit gray ourselves, today. The newness of the hospital experience has worn off quickly. Kathryn has already got herself organized with a system for where she can get easy access to all her essentials (glasses, eye stuff, hair stuff, ear plugs, head phones, tissues, hand wipes, phone chargers and a thousand other important knick-knacks). The transplant unit is a constant hive of activity with repeated tasks of checking Kathryn's pulse, blood pressure, temperature, poking her and prodding her, with people coming in and out to interrupt her with questions. Modesty and privacy have been thrown out the window. I am amazed at how patient and upbeat Kathryn continues to be. We know that her energy will drop a ton over the next week as the conditioning drugs take their toll on her body and her hair falls out and her blood counts drop. For now we both need to keep ourselves immersed in clichés of taking "one day at a time," "baby steps," "focusing on the task at hand," "thinking positive thoughts," and knowing that things will have to get worse before they can get better.

INCARCERATION WITH FRIENDS

Kathryn

July 20, 2014

So here I am on only day 3 (-5 in transplant language) and I'm really feeling the confinement. Having spent quite a bit of time in jail (I was a nurse in the King County Jail for several years – I was never an inmate!), I will say that this place is quieter, less dangerous, and the people have all been kind and helpful. Even so, I totally underestimated what the absence of fresh air would feel like. Luckily, I can at least see it out my window even though I can't smell it or feel that breeze on my face. It's seems unreal to see MY name above a hospital room door. There's a place on my white board to write in a discharge date. When the doctor was in this morning I floated the idea of July 22nd but he didn't go for it.

I wasn't really prepared for the tremendous loss of autonomy that this experience would involve--no purse/wallet, giving up my contacts and great field of vision, losing my hair, having all bodily waste carefully collected and measured each day by people I don't know. I am very lucky to have an excellent caregiver who is prepared to visit me and even do my laundry so that I can have some of my own clothes. Sleeping has been as hard as I was promised it would be--frequent wakings, beeping that only stops if you call somebody, etc. I can tell though that they try hard to minimize sleep disruption. That does count for something and at least I don't have a roommate.

A Patient Care Technician just walked in and asked me where the patient was. I told him I am the patient. I will accept being in the bed with pajamas on when I must, but for now I'm reading by the window. I've had my 2 days of cytoxan and one day of busulfan. So far, so good. Three more to go. Then I have a day of "rest," but they say it really isn't. I don't know what that means. I've been trying to create a welcoming atmosphere for these drugs to prepare my bone marrow for the new cells that I will get on Friday. This week a caring stranger somewhere will be getting injections to rev her body up to make extra cells for me, and I am profoundly grateful. I am also well aware that I will need to feel worse before I can feel better but will try to keep doing as much as I can as I move forward.

Thanks for all the love and care.

Kathryn

MY CAGED AND WOUNDED LIONESS...

Dave

July 21, 2014

Here we are on **Day -4**. Kathryn had her second dose of Busulfan today so she is two thirds of the way through the "bad stuff"... although we remind ourselves that this is really the "good stuff" because it is destroying the bad cells, but also lots of her good cells.

Speaking of cells, Kathryn spends her days padding around in her "cell" looking longingly at the real world outside and more than slightly frustrated at how confined she is. She prowls back and forth in front of the "bars" trying to ignore the injuries that are being inflicted on her through her intravenous line - a toxic chemical soup that acts to make her feel weaker, more nauseated, and less and less able to fight back. She continues to "fight back," however, by force-feeding herself and pounding out the miles along the corridors in the knowledge that this will get harder and harder to do as her blood counts keep going down. Her nurse brought the results of her daily lab work in while I was here today and announced cheerfully, "Your counts keep going down, Kathryn, so that's good!" And of course it is. They need to know that they gave big enough doses of Cytoxan and Busulfan to wipe out her bone marrow to know that the myelofibrosis has been dealt with and her marrow is ready for the new houseguests who will hopefully arrive on Friday (**Day 0**).

While I was at work this morning Kath decided to get her head shaved. Now for all of you with a voyeuristic bent I'm going to have to disappoint you. We are **NOT** going to post those pictures on Caring Bridge, even though I told her that if she let me draw cartoons on her bald pate, and she danced a jig and let me videotape her it could become an overnight sensation and go viral on YouTube, rivaling cute kitten and Corgi videos. Instead you will just need to content yourself with my cool, objective, candid and graphic description... Kathryn looks totally adorable with her head shaved! She looks wa-a-a-ay cuter than the Dalai Lama (and most people would agree that he is pretty darned cute). She also has much better dress sense than most Hare Krishna monks whom I have seen trying to sell me pamphlets on Princes Street in Edinburgh over the years. And I won't insult Kathryn with comparisons to Sinead O'Connor... If Kathryn's head had to stay like this for the rest of her life I wouldn't mind a bit. Her beauty shines from within as bright as ever, like a beacon of love, energy, and grace, drawing in those around her... and like a searchlight penetrating the skies on the darkest of nights with quirky commentaries on the world around her. The sparkle in her eyes just melts my heart as it has done for the past 28 years, and as it will continue to do for many, many, many years to come. It will actually be easier to give her really deep, soothing, effective scalp massages while she is hairless so she may elect to keep her head like this for quite a while.

I won't torture the metaphor any further by saying they have shaved off the lion's mane because for all of you who have spent hours and hours watching Kratts Creatures and Zaboomafoo on Public Television (as Murray and I have done) you already know that lionesses not only do most of the hard work around the Savannah (unlike the complacent and lazy male lions), lionesses don't actually **have** manes. But if you want a lasting vision of Kathryn on **Day -4** just imagine a lioness wearing a flaming gypsy-red head-scarf and staring through the bars of her cage at you... just daring you to take pity on her. She has no time for that. She needs to keep working on her escape plan...

OVER THE HUMP, INTO THE SLUMP

Kathryn

July 22, 2014

Day -3: I now have only one more busulfan infusion to go and I definitely feel it--low counts, weakness, headache, retching, and developing mouth swelling and ulcers that will last until engraftment begins. It's daunting to contemplate how long this road will be, and hard to maintain a sense of humor knowing that I will feel worse and worse before I eventually feel better. This is not a surprise but it's not easy just waiting for the effects to arrive.

A few people have asked about visiting, and I appreciate the offer. Although there are no official visiting hours, as I see my counts approach zero, I'd like to visit with people once I'm considered fit for discharge-

-absolute neutrophil count of 500 and no other big problems. I am taking a LOT of pills to reduce my risk of infection and can't think of any reason to push my luck.

I'm really impressed with the staff here but a combination of no fresh air, no exercise, and no sleep is sure not a recipe for mental or physical health. Hopefully, cytoxan, busulfan, and a transplant will be, in time.

That's it for now - for a while, I'm guessing.

Many thanks for all the good wishes.

Kathryn

CONTINUING CHEMICAL WARFARE

Dave

July 24, 2014

Okay, you may think I am being a bit too melodramatic with that title, and I did say in a previous entry that both Kathryn and I are trying to avoid the oft-used analogy of "fighting" or "battling" cancer for what she is going through. We'd rather think that she is trying to make friends with all these new "toxins" that she is being given and that we can maximize the beneficial effects from them and hope to slip through with as few side effects as possible. But the comparison to chemical warfare is really apt on several different levels. The "big guns" that Kathryn has been given for the past six days, Cyclophosphamide and Busulfan, are alkylating agents and derivatives of nitrogen mustard and related to the mustard gas that caused misery and death during the First World War and more recently in the Middle East.

When I went through Medical School in Edinburgh in the 1970s the Head of the Therapeutics Department was a pompous man called Ronald Girdwood who was fond of name-dropping the various famous colleagues he had worked with over the years.

"As I said to Sir Derrick Dunlop back in 1957... of course he wasn't **Sir** Derrick back in those days... just plain Derrick... now where was I?"

Another of Professor Girdwood's more famous and memorable phrases was to talk about drug side effects like this.

"The more powerful the drug, my boy, the more severe are its side effects... just as the most beautiful roses often have the most wicked thorns. Think of drug side effects as the thorns on the therapeutic rose."

Well, Kathryn-the-gardener is getting a major life lesson on that topic these days. SCCA are being very generous, not only with the quantity of drugs that they are giving her but with the staggering variety - I mean we wouldn't want her body to get bored with just a dozen or so different chemicals. So because one of the possible side effects of Busulfan is causing epileptic seizures they have been giving her a drug called Dilantin to prevent those. But Dilantin causes mental fogginess and some nausea so they are giving Kathryn anti-nausea medication to help with the side effects of the drug they are giving to help with the side effects of yet another drug, and so on...

Kathryn's body is being bathed in an ever-changing chemical soup that will hopefully get her through all this in decent shape. The basic broth still includes a prophylactic anti-viral (acyclovir), an anti-bacterial (Bactrim), and an anti-fungal (fluconazole) along with drugs to protect the liver (ursodiol) and to minimize bone loss (Calcium and Vitamin-D). She had her last dose of Busulfan yesterday but has to get one more day of Dilantin.

Today is euphemistically referred to the "rest day" (or **Day -1**), which is sandwiched between the end of her "conditioning chemo" and the transplant transfusion that she will get tomorrow. However, the term "rest" is a misnomer around here. I have been at her bed since 6:45 a.m. this morning and have so far counted 8 different people "popping in" to poke and prod her, offer helpful suggestions, take her vitals, ask about her bowel movements, offer her medications for nausea or anxiety or pain or...

And now that we are done with the conditioning chemo Kathryn started a new drug at midnight last night. She is now getting a continuous infusion of Tacrolimus added to her soup for the next several weeks. This is a calcineurin inhibitor - a powerful immunosuppressive drug that will hopefully stop Kathryn's body from rejecting the new cells that she will get tomorrow. And then later the Tacrolimus will hopefully prevent (or reduce the severity of) the new cells attacking Kathryn's body (graft-versus-host or GVH disease). Tacrolimus, of course, has its own boatload of potential side effects but we will quietly wait to see which if any she gets and how severe they are.

And so it goes on. One of the many hard things about all of this is that the effects (both good and bad) of many of these drugs are delayed in time. So although she is done with her conditioning drugs (the

Cyclophosphamide and Busulfan) they will continue to exert their powerful effects during the next 2-3 weeks. They are destroying her own bone marrow and immune cells (so her blood counts keep dropping) and will cause increasing amounts of damage and inflammation to the cells that line her mouth, lungs, vagina, and GI tract (a condition called mucositis). Depending on how bad all of that is she may have pain, nausea, diarrhea, difficulty swallowing, fever, and general misery... but not to worry, we have other drugs to give her for each of those symptoms. Yay!

RELIEF FROM MONOTONY

Kathryn

July 25, 2014

As some of you know, I have always had an extremely active dream life. These days, there is more potential for fun and variety during my sleeping hours than during my waking ones. I had quite a good time last night at a Puget Sound Consumers' Co-op (PCC) Cheese Festival. I sampled all kinds of cheese and crackers, covered in cheeses I am now not allowed. As if that wasn't enough fun, I went from there to a Community Festival in north Georgia where I did healthcare work in the Appalachian Mountains with friends Tina and Nancy. I got to listen to old time music while serving guests hot buttery drinks.

Today my cells arrive. I've been told that American cells usually arrive and are infused mid-day but cells coming from Europe usually come about midnight and are infused at 2am. One staff member guessed that mine were coming from Germany but I don't know yet for sure. Offering the potential for a new lease on life, some patients have birthday cakes for this event. I don't have a party planned but Dave will stay with me, and maybe Cameron and Murray if plans change and the infusion is during waking hours. The hours following the infusion require many vital sign checks so sleep may be hard to come by.

I keep thinking of my donor, not only with gratitude but hoping everything is going well for her. I am able to send her an anonymous thank you now but cannot know who she is for a year. I so hope that my family and I can thank her at that time, maybe in person. If she's across the Atlantic, that would make it even more exciting.

Thanks again for all the love and support during this most difficult time in my life.

Love,
Kathryn

A CONVERSATION WITH THE NIGHT VISITORS

Dave

July 26, 2014

A quiet knock on the door at 1:30am announced the arrival of the cells that were to be transferred into Kathryn's body after a careful vetting process that has taken about six months. There was no fanfare, just hushed words of explanation about the process from Emily, the smiling and competent night nurse. Kathryn and I had tried to get some sleep, she in her hospital bed hooked up to the bags of fluid hanging from her ever-present IV pole, me in a recliner chair at her beside. The transfusion was started at 1:41am and took a slow, leisurely trickle through the plastic tubing, through the infusion pump and on towards her central Hickman IV line so that the cells only began to enter Kathryn's body at about 02:00am. Emily stayed with us to monitor Kathryn for fever, hives, changes in pulse or blood pressure, pain, or swelling in her throat. There was none of that, so the transfusion was speeded up and we took a quick photograph to celebrate the moment. Kathryn doesn't feel good about how she looks on account of the bags under her eyes. I, on the other hand, am amazed at how **GOOD** she looks given all the bags that have been hanging at her side and dripping all manner of things into her body for the past eight days!

Some people celebrate this day like it is a new birthday, with cake, candles, kazoos, and songs. We chose to celebrate it quietly with immense gratitude, a big dash of realism, and some sense of foreboding about what might be ahead. There is no going back from here. This gift of life comes with no guarantees. We don't know what kind of future Kathryn will have from here on out.

Many animals, including humans, give birth at night in caves and under bushes, away from the prying eyes of predators. They want this new life to enter the world quietly and unnoticed. That is how Kathryn and I felt last night. I then tried to help Kathryn rest and get back to sleep as best she could. When she was quiet I stood by her bed and watched her new visitors drip slowly into her body, about five million feisty new cells being added to the pulsating river of blood coursing through her body. I decided to have a quiet conversation with them. It went something like this:

"Hello there little cells. I want to thank you from the bottom of my heart as you trickle into the bottom of Kathryn's heart to begin your new journey. It has been a busy week for you, I know, and a very long day. You might be feeling dizzy from being spun around in the centrifuge and a bit jet-lagged from being hurled up into the sky, sent out over Canada and brought back down to SeaTac airport before getting rushed up I-5 to the hospital. Take a deep breath. Kathryn and I are immensely grateful to your previous owner for sharing you with Kathryn. Don't be sad about it. That generous young woman kept lots of your brothers and sisters inside her own body back in New Jersey. So now all of you are protecting TWO incredible women and giving them both your protection and the gift of life.

I'm not sure how to address you properly or what to call you. There aren't very well thought through protocols of etiquette for this situation. You may have noticed that I have an accent. I will speak slowly so that you can maybe understand me better, although if you have spent most of your life in New Jersey then you are probably used to a variety of accents already and people who speak incredibly fast. When I was growing up in Scotland and went to a new school, new kids were always referred to by the name of the village, town, or county where they had come from. So I would hear, "Hey, Mahaar, what did your mammy pack you fur your lunch?" or "Hey, Ayrshire, did you figure out number 5 on last night's Maths homework? Gimme a look, eh?" Now at this point I don't know much about you at all, and we won't know much about your previous owner for twelve months more but I do know that you just came from Montvale, New Jersey. So you hail from the mountains and valleys of The Garden State? Kathryn would approve of all of that. As you will soon find out she loves mountains, valleys, and gardens. I think I'll call you "Jersey." In Scotland the name "jersey" is used to describe a hand-knitted sweater or pullover, something you pull on to protect yourself from the cold, wind, and rain... from the hostile elements in the environment. I like that symbolism, too. You can protect Kathryn from hostile elements in the environment, Jersey.

Let me try to give you some orientation to make it easier for you to get used to your new home. You may notice that you are being accompanied by several big strong chemicals in the liquid whirling along with you around Kathryn's body. One of these is called Tacrolimus. With a name like that I imagine him to be a Roman Centurion. He is there to protect both you and Kathryn from each other, to keep you calm, and to help you both to get along well together. Now I know you will be eager to get to work fighting infections and snuffing out any lingering cancer cells you come across. Feel free to roam around anywhere you like and "do your thing," as they say. Do they use that expression in New Jersey? But for the next couple of weeks you will have enough on your plate just finding the best neighborhood to move into so they have filled Kathryn's blood with Levofloxacin, Fluconazole, and Acyclovir to fight all manner of infections so that you won't have to for a while. Make yourselves at home.

Let me tell you a little bit about Kathryn, which you might find helpful as you are settling in. She is incredibly kind and thoughtful towards others and wishes only the best for all of you, so I hope that you will be nice to her, in return. Please spend your time fighting cancer cells and intruders and leave Kathryn's healthy body alone. I hope you don't mind sudden jolts of movement and bursts of energy. Kathryn tends to jump out of bed in the morning with fierce determination to rush headlong into some new project or other with wild energy and enthusiasm. Just hold on for the ride. She will take you on some amazing adventures.

One last thing, and I can tell you from long experience that this one is tricky... when Kathryn needs to make a decision about something important she always, **always**, does her homework and then comes up with at least three options. She will then ask you what you think is your favorite option. Here's the best advice I can give you. Try to tune in to her and pay attention to the subtle cues and vibes that she is giving off... You may get better at doing that than I am. It definitely takes practice! Whenever you sense which option you think that **she** is leaning towards just keep your demeanor cool and neutral and say, "Hmmm, I think I like this option, what do you think, Kath?" She'll be delighted at how smart you are, and you will have a much happier time afterwards!

So welcome to Kathryn's lovely body, Jersey girls. I hope that she will take you to far-flung places and that she will share wonderful adventures with you for many, many happy years to come.

Your friend,
Dave

WILING AWAY THE HOURS IN A LUXURY EUROPEAN SPA

Dave

July 27, 2014

I hope you will forgive Kathryn and me for having a penchant for gallows humor through all of this. We are constantly impressed (not to mention sobered, subdued, and terrified) at the staggering variety of ways that this process can go wrong and the multitude of ways that you can die during each stage. I may well have to describe some of those in future journal entries so brace yourself. But in all of our reading about potential ways to die they never mention the problem of **dying of boredom...**

Okay, okay, I know that I should now fill a paragraph with politically correct caveats acknowledging that I understand why they have all these rules, why they check up on Kath so often, and "Yes" we are incredibly grateful for everything being done for her. Kathryn has no right to be bored or ungrateful whatsoever. After all, Kathryn's room is a whole lot bigger than the cells at Guantanamo, I am sure, and her jailers (sorry, I mean nurses) are probably much nicer although not always with a better sense of humor. We should be grateful that Kathryn's experience is not unlike spending her days in a luxurious European hotel room. Let me give you a quick tour of her luxury hotel room to make the point so that you can see why she has no reason whatsoever to feel bad about her current situation.

First let's check out the mantelpiece. This is very similar to how yours looks around the holiday season I am sure. There is the festive computer monitor where they document what drugs Kathryn needs. There is a generously wide screen to accommodate the number of drugs that Kathryn has to take. You will also see some holiday latex gloves, a flashlight, antibacterial hand sanitizer, and six (that's right, **SIX**) plastic barf basins. Each of these has a capacity of about one-and-a-half gallons in case you were wondering. There are alcohol swabs, tissues, adhesive tape, a water jug, a regular trash bag and a much more colorful biohazard trash bag, along with tubing and supplies with which to decorate the IV pole. This is just like decorating the Christmas tree at home, really, so just warm your hands by the fireplace and soak up the ambience.

Across the room is Kathryn's powder room area. Here we have mouthwash, gargle, soap, hand-sanitizer, plastic gloves, chlorhexidine wipes (are you spotting a theme here in the hotel room?). Nearby on the wall you will find more electrical outlets than there are on the Control Deck of the Starship Enterprise. These are there to supply the needs of the IV pole, the infusion pumps, the suction pumps, the ventilator, the heart monitor, the blood pressure cuff and about eighteen other brightly colored flashing and beeping machines. Forgive me, I'm getting a bit of a headache. Let's take a trip to the restroom.

First take a look at the welcoming ambience of the restroom door. Please note, "We want you to **CALL** (you idiotic moron!) We don't want you to **FALL!**" The blurred black and white notice to the left of this is there to remind the helpful nurses, nursing students, nursing assistants, and perky and enthusiastic volunteers (who "pop in" singly or in smiling groups at least once an hour) to make sure they ask Kathryn the five "Ps"

Pain - ***What is your pain level?*** Which reminds me of the great scene in The Princess Bride when Wesley is being tortured in The Pit of Despair...

Potty - ***Do you need to use the restroom?*** If so, remember "We want you to **CALL** (you idiotic moron!) We don't want you to **FALL!**"

Position - ***Are you in a comfortable position?*** Kathryn has some very choice rejoinders to this question but usually manages to just smile sweetly and nod her head (which is what they would prefer that you do).

Proximity - ***Is everything you need within reach?*** Ha! That one must be a cruel joke for someone like Kathryn. "No, actually about 99.999% of what I need is a long way outside of this hospital room."

Personal Needs - ***Is there anything else you need?*** Kathryn would bite her tongue over this one except that biting her tongue would be a source of infection, which would create biohazardous bodily fluids. Instead she just sighs. Giving a truthful answer to some of the humor-challenged nurses would just sap too much of Kathryn's energy and since she is, by now, bursting for the bathroom let's go inside.

Note the elegant European touches to the bathroom ambience. The entire floor is tiled and there is enough room in there so that Kathryn could share her decadent and leisurely shower with a friend (wink, wink!). That friend could either be an olive-skinned, hairy-chested Italian gigolo with dreamy eyes, OR... her ever-present IV pole! She gets to choose, which is a pretty good deal if you ask me. Please also notice the grab bars on the walls because in case you have forgotten, "We want you to **CALL** (you idiotic moron!), We don't want you to **FALL!**"

Take note of the UWMC's elegant take on the French bidet. No bodily fluids will go unmeasured! Enough said...

They don't skimp on artwork either in this luxury hotel room. Everywhere you look there are posters which are not only pleasing to the eyes, they also offer helpful and practical hints to prevent you from becoming bored. For example on the lid of the elegant and classy Biohazard Soiled Linen Container is this cute little cartoon. **Are you overfilling me?** Remember, "We want you to **CALL...**"

And finally to keep your spirits up there is a cheerful picture reminding you to disinfect the entire surface of your body at least once an hour. Notice that the cute, smiling, black, bald cartoon character is having a really good time even though her head is no longer attached to the rest of her body (I guess she forgot to **CALL!**). She is luxuriating in a bathtub (which of course no one on the transplant unit is allowed to do but we'll let that one go). She is clearly delighted to be bathing herself, not in boring old Chanel No. 5 parfum, but rather in Eau-de-Chlorhexidine which is much more alluring don't you think?

SLINGS AND ARROWS...

Dave

July 28, 2014

So here we are on **Day +2**. I know that some of you may have been thinking, "Great, her transplant seemed to go well. That wasn't so bad. I guess she just gets steadily better from here on out, right?"

Not exactly.

On the one hand Kathryn is, so far, doing as well or maybe even better than expected but the path forward is extremely tortuous and long. We need to be patient and yet realistic. One way that I do that is to compartmentalize the potential "slings and arrows" that we will face. Some of them are unpleasant, miserable, and painful but are almost certain to occur and so they just need to be suffered until they pass, as they will, in time. Mucositis (a severe inflammation of the cells lining the mouth, guts, lungs and elsewhere) is in this category. Virtually everyone gets it for at least a few days to several weeks. It can be crippling or not-so-bad. There are treatments that alleviate the symptoms and if you hang in there it will eventually go away and you'll feel better.

Then there are more serious problems that can kill you if they are not quickly diagnosed and treated, but most of these **can** be treated. Infections are in this category. The most common sources of these infections for someone like Kathryn are "bugs" living inside her body that are normally kept in check by a healthy immune system but which can run rampant when someone is vulnerable as Kathryn is right now. For the next few weeks Kath has essentially no immune system of her own to defend herself but it will be 10 to 20+ days before "Jersey's" immune system will engraft and start protecting Kathryn.

There is also a third category of "slings and arrows" that are much harder to defend against and cannot be totally treated or cured but can hopefully be contained and subdued before they kill you. Graft-versus-host (GVH) disease is in this category but we are too early in the process to worry about that one today. I may well write about it later.

So today Kathryn felt a little worse. Her energy level was lower, she had some stomach pains like a knot in the center of her guts, and she had diarrhea. Now this could be a manifestation of mucositis in which case it is in category one and we just tough it out. But it could also be an early sign of a very serious infection of the bowels caused by a nasty bacterium called Clostridium difficile (or "C-diff"). They have sent off some of Kath's poop to test it for C-diff but in the meantime we need to take even more precautions. When I arrived to see her late this afternoon I had to wear a gown and gloves before I could enter her room. Kathryn doesn't need to wear those while she is in her European-spa-hotel-room but **does** need to gown and glove up when she leaves her inner sanctum and wanders out into the corridors outside. So imagine, if you will, our heroine trudging through the halls of the transplant unit this evening wearing a sickly yellow gown of the "one-size-fits-no-one" variety, and wrinkly blue plastic gloves pushing her IV pole laden with beeping and flashing infusion pumps and hanging bags of fluids through an obstacle course of food trolleys, X-ray techs, nurses moving beds in and out of other rooms, cleaners polishing the floors, and sleep-deprived doctors logged on to computers lining the hallways. They quickly figured out they would need to get out of Kath's way. She had only done sixteen laps so far today and was determined to get to twenty before she could quit and start "relaxing" for the evening.

After our laps Kath got to take off her gown and gloves to go back into her room but I had to gown and glove up to join her. So there we sat for a totally relaxed and comfortable evening together, just hanging out, kicking back, and shooting the breeze about the lazy carefree days stretching ahead of us...

In Shakespeare's famous soliloquy from Hamlet he contemplates what it means to take action when you are faced with ill fortune in life.

"Whether 'tis nobler in the mind to suffer the slings and arrows of outrageous fortune, or to take arms against a sea of troubles, and by opposing end them?"

Well, we are in for a "sea of troubles," that's for

sure. Some of these troubles will just need to be suffered with as much stoicism, grace, and patience as we can muster. With others we will need to fight them with great courage and determination.

Since our evening had a surreal, comical, and hopeless feel to it we decided to take our minds off our current troubles by escaping into another comedic and philosophical masterpiece. We watched (for maybe the tenth time!) ***The Big Lebowski*** by the Coen brothers. It lifted my spirits to see Kathryn almost choking on her dinner because of her laughter. For those of you who have seen this movie (which is definitely on my top ten list of all time greats, which may say something about me...) you will remember that in this brilliant farce things go from bad to worse to unbelievably-impossible-he'll-never-get-out-of-this... but eventually everything actually **does** turn out okay. At the end of the movie Jeff Bridges just shrugs and smiles.

"The Dude abides, man."

Today I take some comfort in that sentiment. The Dude abides, man. Let's see what **Day +3** brings...

A QUICK SIGH OF RELIEF... FOR NOW

Dave

July 29, 2014

Just a quick update today since I am feeling weary and tired. Kathryn's C. difficile test came back negative so we can stop doing the gown and glove routine for now. Her other labs continue their predictable decline (in red cells, white cells and platelets). She had another small blood transfusion last night (they only give a single unit of packed cells each time her hematocrit dips below 26). Today she felt a little better, in terms of energy and sore mouth and sore throat and sore butt and... okay TMI for some of you, I know! This is now **Day +3** so we are a day closer to engraftment. She has kept all her food down, has done 22 laps and has had a nice boring uneventful day.

Kath is appreciative of the food here at the

hospital. It is edible and is prepared in ways that are safe for those on an immunosuppressive diet. But it is rather boring and repetitive so I brought in something that I prepared at home for a bit of variety. It was a simple avocado, mango, and bean salad but took about three times as long as it normally would to prepare because all the prep surfaces and knives and plates and bowls need to be cleansed with bleach before you start, every piece of fresh fruit or vegetable has to be washed thoroughly under cold running water before you even cut into it and again once you have chopped it up. Each can of pinto or cannellini beans needs to be washed on the outside in hot soapy water and then get rinsed in warm un-soapy water before putting a bleach-sanitized can opener anywhere near it. After using the can opener on one can of food it needs to be re-sanitized in bleach, and then rinsed before you can open the next can. Every single lettuce leaf needs to be thoroughly washed under cold running water and then shaken dry, and so on. Luckily Kathryn thought it tasted pretty good (and did not taste of bleach!) so I'll call that a success.

Here's to more uneventful days ahead.

A FIELD TRIP!

Kathryn

July 30, 2014

Other than contact with family and friends, the highlight of my week is bound to be the field trip that I took to radiology for a chest X-ray. That meant getting off the transplant unit (!) I thought maybe we could make a leisurely stroll out of it but that's not how it works. I was bundled into a wheel chair, wrapped up in a blanket and delivered to the radiology desk by a friendly guy named Ben. I was pretty sure the trip wouldn't involve any fresh air but I did get out of here and saw some new territory for an hour. For the return trip, I was put into the wheel chair again and parked somewhere to wait for the courier. I felt like a UPS parcel waiting to be picked up and delivered.

Speaking of medical tests, I feel compelled to apologize to any of you readers who might be squeamish. Healthcare people are overrepresented among our friends so we think nothing of describing things like my C-diff culture and other bodily details. I have a sense of all the big and small problems I could have when I am questioned regularly about all aspects of my GI tract, rashes, itching, pain, swelling etc. Luckily, my body is behaving pretty well so far.

One of my favorite Medical Assistants is a young man from Eritrea named Teages. He is always cheerful, polite, and helpful. I was asking him last night about his path from Eritrea to my bedside. He came here a few years ago and drove a cab for 3 years but wanted to challenge himself. He has now gotten trained to do work that he finds much more rewarding. At one point in our conversation he said, "We have to be sick. It's our life. If all the time we good (big expansive hand gesture) we know nothing." Seems in his young life he already understands the value of suffering.

Medically, I am told things are going better than they often do. I can't help but think all the prayers and positive energy sent our way by all of you have something to do with it. My labs all look good and the attending today said he sees very little sign of toxicities from the treatment at this point. Given what the treatment has been, I'm really grateful for that. As if that wasn't enough, I have the most excellent, attentive, industrious, and good-humored caregiver I could ever want.

Thanks to all of you for the continued support in this long haul.

Sweet dreams.

Kathryn

SLIPPING QUIETLY THROUGH THE DAYS

Dave

July 31, 2014

So here we are on **Day +5** with Kathryn feeling remarkably well all things considered. Yes, her blood counts remain frighteningly low but this is absolutely what everyone looking after her wants and expects. In fact we would all worry if her counts were not dropping. Kath continues to have only very mild GI discomfort, is eating well, and is doing her part with typical vigor and determination. She gargles with saline mouthwash more often than they recommend, forces herself to eat nutritious food even when she doesn't feel hungry, drinks plenty of water even though it means more trips to the bathroom, and does three times as many laps around the transplant unit as anyone else. For this she gets the kind of comments she has gotten her whole life:

"Wow, sister, you is MOVING!"

"We all need to get out of your way, I can see that."

"Heads up, she's coming through. Lord, you are burning up the floor, young lady!"

For those of you who know Kathryn you know that she is **not** trying to show off or to impress anyone. That is just the way her body moves. It is when she slows down that I get concerned.

I sat by Kathryn's bedside for several hours during the day yesterday. The Wi-Fi reception is excellent so I can easily deal with work-related e-mails and minor "crises" using my laptop. Kathryn tracks on when she is due for checks on her vital signs, blood tests, lab results, when the cleaners will interrupt (she also knows their names and engages them in conversation about how **their** lives are going), when the nursing shift changes, when they ought to be emptying her toilet... She carefully sets out her many pills for the day into small piles of those that need to be taken once a day or twice a day, with food or on an empty stomach, which ones should not be taken with which other ones, and then she meters them out appropriately throughout the day.

Kathryn tries to break up her day with activity, rest, and "entertainment." We listened to about 45 minutes of National Public Radio together but that was as much as we could take. Let me summarize the state of the world for those of you who may have been too busy to be paying attention recently:

There are a who-o-o-o-o-ole lot of people in the world who are angry and unhappy and want to wreak violence, hatred, and death on other nearby people who, I have to say as I look on from afar, look virtually identical in appearance, lifestyle, and in their hopes and aspirations to the other group who hate them, but apparently they believe **slightly** different versions of various ancient received "truths" and so for that reason they are to be vilified and destroyed. This appears to be true whether they are reporting from Northern Ireland, Iraq, Syria, or Africa. Tolerance is nowhere to be seen... Of course in reality there are billions of people around the world who **are** kind, thoughtful, tolerant, and helpful to those around them but apparently that is not newsworthy.

Kathryn and I amused ourselves by getting an alternative take on the news by watching recent clips of ***The Daily Show*** with ***Jon Stewart*** and ***Last Week Tonight*** with ***John Oliver***. John Oliver did a wonderful expose of the multibillion dollar snake-oil (a.k.a. unproven and unregulated vitamin and supplement) industry as peddled by Oprah and Dr. Oz. Hilarious and sad all at the same time.

But ever the multitasker, Kathryn had a hard time sitting still during all of this. So she got out her color-coded-stretchy-large-sized-exercise-rubber-bands and tied one end to various items in her room: her tray table, bathroom door handle, ceiling light fixtures, her long-suffering visitor, the TV monitor or IV pole. She then attached the other end of the stretchy bands to her ankle or wrist... it was all very relaxing for me, as you can imagine. Kathryn then stretched and grunted to her heart's content while issuing brief commentaries such as:

"*Polite-expletive* this is boring!"

or

"I am so sick of using these *not-so-polite-expletive* stretchy bands. I would so-o-o-o-o much prefer to quit right now... but I need to do ten more reps and then tie it to my other ankle. Oh, hey, it's about time for me to call and order my dinner. Gotta keep choking down that nutrition..."

And so the days pass. I will continue to stay by your side, Kath, but will try to learn when to keep out of your way. We are definitely not wishing our lives away but here's to slipping quietly into **Day +6** and beyond...

MORE ABOUT PLATELETS (AND LATIN!) THAN YOU EVER WANTED TO KNOW

Dave

August 1, 2014

Spoiler Alert: *For those of you who prefer the warmer and fuzzier journal entries about how Kathryn is doing and how we are feeling about this very long and uncertain journey you might want to stop reading this right now. Not everyone finds platelets to be interesting, let alone warm and fuzzy, although I think that they* **are** *all of those things, both literally and figuratively. Kathryn and I are trying to understand as much as we possibly can about the science behind what is happening to her body. We want to appreciate the strategies behind her treatment options and to challenge the team at SCCA to explain them to us when those strategies don't make sense to us.*

Today Kathryn's platelet count fell below 7,000, which is a really low number. That is both good (because it means that they gave her an effectively BIG dose of conditioning chemotherapy) and bad (because when the platelets are below 10,000 you are at risk of having a catastrophic bleed into your brain or other important organs). So they gave Kathryn a platelet transfusion this morning along with a blood transfusion and a boatload of other drugs.

So let me tell you some interesting things about platelets... along with some editorial comments about the medical profession! The healthy bone marrow makes three main types of cells: red blood cells, white blood cells and platelets. Some would say that platelets are not technically cells since they have no nucleus. However, the cells that make platelets **do** have nuclei. They are great big (MEGA) cells that live in the bone marrow and so they are called megakaryocytes. They crank out loads and loads of platelets. Platelets are also called thrombocytes because they are "cells" (-cytes) that help us to form clots (thrombus). When everything is working properly millions of these happy little thrombocytes whizz around in your warm blood waiting to be helpful. If you cut yourself and start to bleed the platelets zoom in like Medic-One and are first on the scene to help out. They change shape, become fuzzier (I kid you not), stick to each other and help to form a clot to stop the bleeding. This is a truly helpful and miraculous process when it all works properly as it did for most of Kathryn's life. But then about ten years ago something went wrong inside Kathryn's bone marrow and she started making too many platelets.

At first the doctors thought Kathryn's problem

was only making too many platelets. Now when doctors don't understand why something is happening they don't want to look stupid. So they use a complicated Latin code language to describe it. They can then hide behind incomprehensible words, sound smarter, and charge more... it is a time-honored tradition in medicine! I mean how well would it go if a patient went to see her doctor and he just shrugged and said,

"Well Mrs. Smith I'm afraid that your body is making way too many platelets and I really don't know why."

"Huh? Well you're not very smart. I think I'll go find somebody else to treat me."

But how much better would it go if the doctor stroked his bow-tie thoughtfully, looked at the patient with his sad, dreamy, intelligent blue eyes and said,

"Well Mrs. Smith I'm afraid that you have a very vexing, but fascinating case of Essential Thrombocytosis."

"Wow, that sounds serious! I'm glad I've got someone as smart as you looking after me."

"Of course you are, my dear, now just write me a large check and leave it at the front desk on your way out."

You see how much more effective it is when we use Medico-Latin-speak! **ET** (which stands for Essential Thrombocytosis and not the Extra Terrestrial even though it means that the person's body is acting in a very alien way!) simply means that the person's bone marrow makes way too many platelets. A normal number is about 250,000 in every milliliter of blood. When Kathryn's bone marrow was at its peak of crazy overproduction her bone marrow poured out well over 1,500,000 in every milliliter. That can be bad for two reasons. As you might expect too many platelets might mean that your body gets **too** good at clotting. You might form clots all over the veins and arteries in your body causing heart attacks, strokes, and other damage. That is all true. Funnily enough when your platelet numbers get that high you also run the risk of bleeding. Why? Because those gazillions of platelets that are cranked out of your revved up bone marrow just rush around like irresponsible teenagers and don't function normally or do anything useful to help you out.

It was because of the increased risk of both clotting and bleeding over the past ten years that Kathryn was treated with hydroxyurea to try to keep her platelets in the 200,000-300,000 range where they ought to be.

But Kathryn's bone marrow wasn't content to only make too many platelets; it was an overachiever and decided to make too many red cells too! The fancy Medico-Latin-speak for that condition is Polycythemia Rubra Vera (or **PRV**). "Poly" means **too many,** "-cyt-" means **cells,** "-hemia" means **in the blood.** "Rubra" tells us that they are **red** cells. And "Vera" means **truly** (and is not thrown in there to honor the doctor's favorite housekeeper called Vera!) So the translation is that "This patient truly makes too many red cells in her blood!" You might think that adding the word "vera" is a pompous affectation but it is not. We use this word to indicate that the overproduction of red cells is truly bad, unhelpful, overproduction. That distinguishes PRV from other situations where a person's **healthy** bone marrow increases its production of red cells but is trying to be helpful. For example if someone smokes and trashes their lungs they may not be able to suck enough oxygen into their body. Oxygen is carried by the red blood cells so that person's body tries to help out by making more red cells to grab onto all the oxygen that it can. They are said to have secondary polycythemia (because it occurred in response to something else such as not being able to suck in enough oxygen).

So Kathryn's revved up bone marrow used to make too many platelets **AND** too many red blood cells. It also decided to make too many fibroblasts. Those are cells that help to form scar tissue. As the scar tissue built up in Kath's bone marrow it left less and less room to make platelets and red and white cells which is why her counts started dropping last year. Her platelets have hovered around 60-100,000 until she got flattened with her conditioning chemotherapy starting fifteen days ago. The platelet levels have been dropping steadily ever since and today reached 7,000.

In summary, over the past decade Kathryn's lovely body has had to cope with platelet counts that have varied from over one-and-a-half-million to under seven thousand. Today's platelet transfusion should raise the counts to safer levels for a few days. In the meantime we will keep waiting for "Jersey" to start kicking in. Of the 14 million or so stem cells that were transfused from Jersey we hope that a couple of million of them will decide to turn into megakaryocytes and start producing platelets. We also hope that Jersey has read the story of Goldilocks and the Three Bears. We want Jersey to produce an amount of platelets that is not too many and not too few but a quantity that is ju-u-u-ust right!

NO MORE SLIPPING QUIETLY

Dave

August 3, 2014

This has been a rough weekend. We are now well into week three of Kathryn's hospital stay. It is 17 days since the heavy doses of conditioning chemotherapy were started. Her doctors have been very surprised at how little this has all been affecting Kathryn but warned that things could change in a hurry. Yesterday they did. Kathryn's cell counts are at rock bottom. She officially has no neutrophils (white cells) whatsoever. Zero. Without taking intense infection precautions and giving her prophylactic infusions of antibacterial, antiviral and antifungal drugs that situation is incompatible with life. Unfortunately they can't give transfusions of white cells... well they can but they don't do much good because of the way white cells behave. All that is to be expected, of course, but it doesn't make it any less scary. When the white cells are this low you can get a fever for no apparent reason but since it **could** represent a bad infection we may have lots more gown-and-glove routines, and more blood cultures in our near future.

More problematic is that mucositis has finally declared itself with a vengeance. Kathryn not only has nausea, gut ache, abdominal pain, pain and itching around her bottom end but she now has significant mouth sores. In typical "Kathronian" fashion when the nurse and physician's assistant looked into her mouth and said,

"Wow, you've got some sores in there, right enough. How do you feel? How much pain do you have?"

Kathryn responded without a trace of sarcasm. "Mmmm it's pretty painful, but not too bad, I suppose. I only feel it when I swallow... or chew... or speak. It's bearable if I just sit here quietly and breathe... so long as I don't breathe too deeply."

The on-call doc was very nice and very experienced and convinced Kathryn that you don't get Brownie points (and don't get better any quicker) by being a stoic and suffering in silence so she has been started on **PCA** which means a Patient Controlled Administration of morphine. She has a little remote control gadget with a button that she can push, but no more often than once every six minutes. Every time she pushes the button the pump beeps and delivers a dose of morphine right into her bloodstream. Now some of you may be thinking,

"Sweet! Sign me up for that bad boy and I'll just sail through the rest of this in a nice fog!"

As you can imagine that is not how Kathryn feels about it. For someone who would rather be sleeping under the stars out in the woods in almost complete silence and who hates flashing lights, beeping noises and who watches virtually no television Kathryn is becoming surrounded by intrusive beeping, flashing robotic machines and more remote controllers than she knows what to do with (the one to raise and lower her bed, the one to turn on the TV, the one to call the nurse, and now the one to give herself six minutes of partial relief from her mouth misery).

After a night of very little sleep Kath got up this morning to take her shower and get back out into the halls to get her laps in so that she can try to keep her strength up so that her blood will keep moving to minimize fluid build up and blood clot formation. With typical understated brevity she simply commented:

"This thing is a lot heavier to shove around today so I guess it is an even better workout of my arms and legs!"

Today is also **Day +8** so we continue to wait for the new stem cells to begin to do their "good things" by producing new cells that will hopefully heal up the mucositis. In the meantime Kathryn will try to grin and bear it... although she has to be careful not to grin too widely or it hurts like hell.

RETURN OF THE FOG

Kathryn

August 4, 2014

I may not be writing for a while since I've been encouraged to use morphine liberally to get through the next week or so. I really hate the drugs that mess with my mind but had to use them last week and have to again now. The worst of it is the stomachache and mouth ulcers and swelling. Since I can't talk or chew or eat, I will be started on IV nutrition later today or tomorrow. Eighteen days of sleep deprivation of course makes everything seem worse.

As I think about all the other people on this unit, I imagine all kinds of different temperaments, levels of education, levels of support. Some of you know that I am a curious person and I have a lot of questions in almost any situation. I desperately want to go door to door and find out how other people are coping with this most difficult treatment plan. Since psychological support really isn't built into this process, it seems like it might be a good idea for patients to share survival strategies with one another. For me, it's been helpful to structure my days around my small activities--shower, dress in street clothes, do laps, a bit of reading if I can, music and resistance bands etc. I'd sure like to gather tips for coping from other patients experiencing the same things.

Most days Dave and I are able to accept that, whether we like it or not, this is the path we have to walk. We have some down days but it only adds to our suffering to imagine what might have been this year. As we have told the kids throughout their lives, when adversity comes our way we have two basic choices--deal with it well or badly. We are giving it our best.

This experience gives me such a sense of taking my place in history. In 2014, the possibility of a cure lies in a giant blast of chemotherapy followed by very severe side effects. As hard as it is to believe, all of what I'm experiencing is part of the plan. The doctor told me again this morning that I'm lucky my mucositis didn't hit a week ago and that I couldn't be doing any better. It may not be too many years before the medical community will look back in disbelief at what they put people through for treatment in 2014. I have described this treatment as both barbaric and miraculous and I am right in the middle of the barbaric part. Let's get on with the miracle.

Thanks for all the love and care in this marathon adventure.

Love,
Kathryn

P.S. Just to be sure I'm not selling SCCA or the Transplant unit short, psychological and spiritual support are both available but it requires asking to speak with someone. I think they are beginning a study looking at having that be a more integral part of pre-transplant and during transplant care.

I want any of you who may need such services to know that the care at SCCA and here has been totally top-notch. I am lucky to live in a city where this was available to me. It also means that for the 4-month treatment plan I get to go home after this instead of to a temporary apartment. Yay.

SHRINKING, NOT SHRIVELING

Dave

August 5, 2014

It is now 19 days since Kathryn was admitted to the UWMC transplant unit and this is **Day +10** since her stem cell infusion. As I chronicle the many steps along this journey I am trying to avoid clichés and platitudes. I want to share honestly what it feels like for me without suffocating everyone with excruciating medical details or interminable descriptions of how miserable this all is for Kathryn. If I were to channel my long-dead Scottish grandmother I wouldn't say anything at all:

"If you can't say anything nice, then don't..."

Another more contemporary American source also restrains me from oversharing the gory details of Kathryn's day-to-day reality. My good friend Matt

(Handley) and I have a colleague at work whom we both admire tremendously. Greg Simon is a psychiatrist who has a great international reputation for the research he has done to improve the treatment for people with depression. He has pioneered new systems of care to make it easier to identify people who have severe depression. The goal is to get them onto appropriate treatment sooner, make sure that they stay on their treatment and get it adjusted to minimize side effects so that more of them feel better and recover faster. But Greg often shocks the medical students, residents, and junior colleagues when he shadows and mentors them as they interview patients. After just a couple of minutes of conversation when the young doctor and the patient are just warming up with detailed descriptions of misery and sadness Greg will interrupt and say,

"So do you think that this lady is depressed?"

"Absolutely!"

"Good. Then let's move on to discuss treatment options with her. **Prolonging the tale of woe is not therapeutic!"**

That is an important lesson to learn as a clinician... or a patient. Kathryn and I recognize this and certainly don't want to wallow in our current day-to-day miseries, linger on the unpleasant details or to prolong the tale of woe. To use up all of my clichés in one sentence we both know that right now we just need to:

"... dig down deep, suck it up, tough it out, hang in there, and never give up because the only way to get past this is to go through it..."

There, that feels better, and at least I managed to avoid using any overt sporting or warfare metaphors!

As Kathryn's day-to-day realities become more

uncomfortable and painful I am struck with how much it feels like the boundaries of her world keep shrinking and shrinking. We are hunkered down in the lowest level of Maslow's hierarchy focusing on shelter, safety from harm, clean air, clean water and some nutritional sustenance. What constitutes success, or something positive, or pleasure gets narrower and smaller and more inward focused.

Success is getting out of bed in the morning when you'd rather curl up under the covers and blubber, taking a shower in tepid water that irritates the skin, forcing yourself into street clothes to plod the interminable halls that smell of floor polish, vomit, and disinfectant.

Something positive is not wincing in pain every time you swallow or turn over in bed. It is managing to produce at least one well-formed poop every day that isn't liquid, itchy, or painful.

Pleasure is lying in the fetal position with a heating pad on your aching belly listening to some loving person read to you from a book of short stories or poems or a chapter from an adventure story that lets you escape from your miserable confinement to the windswept tundra and breathtaking desolation of the Alaskan wilderness. It is getting through fifteen minutes without the intrusion of piercing alarms and flashing lights. It is getting a nurse on the night shift who has a shred of thoughtfulness and a sense of humor instead of the one whose never-ending refrain of "Now is there anything else I can do for you, Kathryn?" has all the sincerity of the "Have-a-Nice-Day" delivered by the garage attendant.

Not everything about Kathryn's current life is shrinking, of course. The number of bags that they hang on her IV pole keeps growing! For those of you keeping score at home we hit our all time record a couple of nights ago. SEVEN different bags were all running at the same time; some big, others small, some clear, some cloudy, others colored. We had saline, magnesium, tacrolimus, levofloxacin, acyclovir, platelets AND morphine. It was very exciting. They were piggybacked onto each other and threaded through four different infusion pumps with the tubing looking like a deranged chef's alien spaghetti recipe. And we are told that they may need to add another transfusion of red cells and some parenteral nutrition (a slurry of amino acids, glucose, vitamins, proteins and essential fats dripped directly into Kathryn's heart) so we might even beat our record and get up to NINE simultaneous infusions tonight. Perhaps we should be calling the folk at the Guinness Book of Records.

But although the boundary of Kathryn's current day-to-day world is shrinking it is not shriveling. All of this is reversible. Our hopes and our dreams are not shrinking; the challenges that we have for each other and ourselves are not getting smaller. The adventures that we plan to have and the number of people we plan to help to laugh and thrive and grow in the future keeps getting bigger and bolder. We may have to postpone and delay some of those dreams for a while yet but our imagination and spirit keeps expanding.

Bring on **Day +11.**

THE JERSEY GIRLS KICK IN!

Kathryn

August 7, 2014

I think of my new cells as "Jersey girls" because they are from a young woman in New Jersey. I have tried to develop a friendly relationship with them from the start, and talk to them daily.

As miraculous as it seems, my new cells from Jersey have started off with a bang and I am now producing neutrophils! After having ZERO for several days, yesterday I had 140, but we wanted to be sure and today I have 380. (The normal range per microliter is roughly 2,500-7,000 so I have a ways to go) We've read that we should expect to see cells 14-28 days after transplant and I'm at Day 12, so we are thrilled to maybe have my hospital stay shortened. We were desperately hoping for this part to go well because not having neutrophils is incompatible with life.

While my family and I celebrate my neutrophils, I feel compelled to write just a little bit about them so that you might celebrate yours. Neutrophils make up about 40-60% of your white blood cells and are one of the first responders in protecting you against infection. They circulate throughout your body in your blood but then actually travel through tissue as they are deployed to areas of injury. They respond to chemical signals from the site of the injury within minutes and can even send for back up help if needed.

As a concrete example, I noticed a small scratch on my arm 2 days ago, cause for worry if you have no neutrophils. My doctor said we wouldn't do anything immediately since it looked clean and my cells should be going to work before long. He explained that if I started producing neutrophils, it would get redder--part of the desired inflammatory response to healing a cut. Sure enough, twenty-four hours later the Jersey girls came through! My scratch is now redder, not infected, and showing signs of beginning to heal.

Although I have always been fascinated by the human body, I have been guilty of taking for granted all the things that work smoothly on any given day, often without my awareness. I forget to be thankful that I wake up most mornings without pain, I can roll over and hug my dear husband, see the sun coming through the window. I know I still have some big hurdles to clear in my transplant treatment, but this experience will leave me a little less apt to take for granted the things that are going **right**.

Dave and I get some training tomorrow about

managing at home and, if our luck continues, will be out of here before the weekend is over!

Love to all of you,
Kathryn

HEADED HOME!

Kathryn

August 9, 2014

I am thrilled to say that tomorrow will probably be my last day here, for now anyway. The miracle of new cell production continues with all my counts rising. To be eligible for discharge, your counts have to be OK and you have to be eating and drinking and free of IVs and serious symptoms. I am aware of how quickly things change here but am hoping I will still be OK for discharge tomorrow. I am grateful to the staff here for the excellent care I have received but I do hope I don't see them again anytime soon.

There are many "milestones" in this four-month to a year treatment plan. Dave and I feel like we don't spend a lot of time celebrating each one because we are acutely aware of what to worry about next. Now that we know the new cells are working, I am being monitored closely for graft versus host disease (GVHD). Dave wrote a little bit about this earlier. It's when the new cells (the graft) recognize me (the host) as foreign and begin attacking healthy organs and tissue.

The acute form happens during the first 3-4 months after transplant and can have major effects on the GI tract, as well as the skin and liver. The chronic form can arise any time after the first 3 months or so and can last for several years. It also affects the GI tract and frequently the skin, eyes, mouth, and other organs.

Both forms of GVHD can be unpleasant and dangerous so we just have to hope that if I get it (80% likely) that it will be mild--in part because the treatment has serious side effects and how much treatment I need depends on how bad it is. Some providers believe the ideal situation is a little bit of graft-versus-host-disease because then the cells might recognize any returning cancer cells and mop them up, hopefully without doing serious or life-threatening damage to other body parts.

It is a challenge sometimes to go forward with optimism when we know as much as we do about the likelihood of more difficulties just around the corner. We are trying to take a day at a time and to make sure we have a bit of pleasure and a good laugh each day. Although we are not happy about the reason we will both be at home over the next couple of months, we will relish the time together.

The support of all of you fortifies our spirits and helps us carry on as we plan for the worst and hope for the best. As hard as this is, we knew it would be difficult and we also know that it is my only chance at living for more than a year or two.

So far, I have been very lucky with how it's all

gone. My whole family really appreciates the love and encouragement from afar.

Love to all of you,
Kathryn

A FEW FIRST IMPRESSIONS

Dave

August 11, 2014

Early morning, **Day +16**, Kathryn is still asleep. This journal entry will need to be short because the realities of my caregiving responsibilities are weighing heavily on me right now. Laundry, food prep, preparing our schedule for the day (temperature check, morning pills, shower, figuring out the new infusion pump, IV fluids, lab and clinic appointments...). All of it is a labor of love, but labor nevertheless. I have so many thoughts and reflections to share... on what the "new normal" is going to look like and feel like... on how quickly (or slowly) Kathryn's life and horizons can start to expand... on new appreciations for "simple things" which aren't really simple at all... but all of those will need to wait. I have chopping boards to bleach and pajamas to take out of the washer and put in the dryer, as well as other mundane but delightful things before KC is awake.

After numerous bureaucratic discharge hiccups yesterday I was finally able to get Kath home from the hospital at about 6:15pm. Highlights of the evening included watching Kath's face light up as she saw how big many of the garden plants had gotten in the past 24 days, seeing her breathe deeply from the fresh air on the deck, holding her as she sobbed during the sunset over the Kitsap peninsula, having a bowl of warm soup while sitting at the table that was covered in a real tablecloth, feeling that adorable and familiar warm body gently breathing beside me during the quiet night of uninterrupted sleep. Slipping out of bed early so that Kath can sleep until she wakes without being prodded or poked...

More to come.

REFLECTIONS ON AN EVER-CHANGING "NORMAL"

Dave

August 12, 2014

What's in a word? Kathryn and I have heard the word "**normal**" used a lot in recent months.

"It's normal to be anxious about getting a bone marrow transplant."

"Nausea and vomiting are normal with the conditioning drugs that you're getting."

"Insomnia is normal here in the transplant unit."

"You've got mouth sores? Oh, that's normal with mucositis - I'm surprised yours is not worse and didn't come on sooner."

And the number of times we have heard this daunting comment has been ominous:

"Don't expect to get your old life back after the bone marrow transplant. You'll just need to get used to **your new normal.**"

In most of these sentences the word "normal" is being used to mean what is to be "expected," of course.

"Well, under these (highly abnormal!) circumstances you can expect anxiety, nausea, vomiting, insomnia, mouth sores..."

And the use of the phrase "your new normal" seems like code language for an unspecified but diminished quality of life.

I have to say that almost nothing about our life has seemed normal for the past year. It felt abnormal and worrisome that Kathryn's blood counts kept dropping towards the end of last year despite lowering the dose and finally stopping hydroxyurea altogether. It felt abnormal to be given false reassurance about this and then be told that Kathryn's bone marrow biopsy looked very abnormal indeed. We got very different messages about how treatable her myelofibrosis would be, how likely it might be that they could find a "perfect" match for her, or how likely it would be that her body could withstand the preferred full myeloablative conditioning regimen. We learned that uncertainty, mixed messages, and differing opinions were all "normal" under these circumstances.

During the waiting period our "normal" daily routines changed considerably and during Kathryn's 24 days in the UWMC transplant unit the "normal" activities that revolved around her changed dramatically. A total lack of privacy became "normal." Meeting a never-ending stream of well-intentioned strangers was "normal." Accepting infusions of poison and handfuls of pills and learning to tolerate their side effects was "normal." Losing your hair, feeling constant bodily discomfort and mental fatigue was all to be expected as "normal." But what an alien kind of normal it has been.

One of our favorite possessions is a 1983 edition of ***Webster's Unabridged Encyclopedic Dictionary of the English Language***. It sits on a little table in our living room beside a table lamp so that any time one of us hears an unfamiliar word (on the radio, in a book, or newspaper, or out of someone's mouth) and one of us asks, "What does that mean?" we go and look it up and share it with each other. Even in these days of Google and Wikipedia we still use Webster's if we're at home. It is fun to look at nearby words or the neat old-fashioned black and white illustrations on the page. So how does Webster's define ***normal*** on page 983 (a page that also contains Norfolk, North Borneo, and a map of the coast of Normandy, by the way!).

normal *adj.* 1. conforming to the standard or the common type; usual; not abnormal; regular; natural. 2. serving to fix a standard.

(And then there are two psychological definitions which I know will amuse our dear friend Julie G)

3. *Psychol.* a. approximately average in any psychological trait as intelligence, or emotional adjustment. b. free from any mental disorder; sane

In truth, during these past few difficult months and weeks the most constantly normal thing in my life has been Kathryn. Her attitude of endless curiosity, her relentless questioning of those around her to understand what was being done to her and why has been normal. Her patience and her determination have been unchanged by the ordeal. Her sense of humor, while sorely tested at times, has remained normal. The light in her eyes has never wavered. Not for one second did she indicate that going through this was the wrong decision or that giving up was an option. She was never "out of it," and her personality or attitude never changed. She has remained entirely and delightfully "normal." I know that I am somewhat biased but to me the "normal" Kathryn Crawford is not fully or accurately described by Webster's rather bland definitions.

So here on **Day +17** our "normal" four mile walk through the Loop Trail of Discovery Park looked and felt a little different since Kathryn needed to protect herself more than usual from sun exposure and had to carry a little shoulder pack containing one liter of normal saline plus magnesium along with the infusion pump that is pushing it into her central line. But in many ways, as we shared the smells and sights of the woods, and chatted about the latest adventures of our kids and grandkids the whole experience felt really great, just like it always does.

There may well be setbacks ahead, but for now, that walk felt really, really, delightfully, wonderfully **normal**.

OH, THE BREEZES...

Kathryn

Aug 14, 2014

I am now onto day 4 at home and it is wonderful to be here with my people, my garden, and my own bed. I want to thank Gabriella Moller (The Cottage Gardener) and Zan for sprucing up the garden for my welcome home. It's a jumble of color and good cheer. I LOVE our garden and will not be able to work in it for a full year so I really appreciate her expert and artistic help.

I was surprised by some of the things I missed most in the hospital. One of them was feeling a breeze on my skin. I could see leaves fluttering outside my window but not feel a thing. We live on a hill and get nice breezes in the afternoon. I also missed savoring a cup of coffee in my Marble Canyon mug. Being "off leash" for most of the day is terrific. In the hospital, with the exception of 30 free minutes for a shower, I had to tow around my IV pole and bags 24/7. Now I get an IV for 5 hours/day and have it in a backpack so it doesn't keep me from being active.

Dave and I are both surprised at how busy we seem to be in these early days at home. He is cooking me delicious, nutritious food 3 times per day and all items of linen and clothing are single use for now--lots of loads of washing. He is also attending to the garden day-to-day since I can't. I really don't know how I would ever get through this without such a loving, attentive, and good-humored caregiver.

The hospitalization was incredibly difficult but we did know it was time limited. We are now aware of needing to develop some new coping strategies as we face the uncertainties related to graft-versus-host-disease and other complications over the coming year. Since I am very likely to get GVHD, our hope is that it will be mild and not life threatening. I had my first outpatient appointment on Monday and we were encouraged to have my new doctor say that if things go well early (they certainly have), they are more apt to go well later. Dave and I, on the other hand, were worried that we might be using up all of our good luck at the beginning. As always, there are no guarantees. Meanwhile, Dave and I are very much savoring our time together and being at home doing some of our regular things. We hope that a year from now I am feeling relatively well and we feel like our life horizons are expanding a bit.

I am REALLY sick of talking about my body but my body has served me well so far and I will continue to do what I need to to take care of it. My Jersey girls continue to do an energetic job of providing me with better blood counts than I've had for a year. I will spare you a litany of my various symptoms and expect that Dave and I will be writing here somewhat less often as we enter the very long, but less dramatic, part of the journey. We will continue to post updates from time to time whether things are going well or badly.

Thanks again to all of you for the ongoing encouragement and support. I don't underestimate the role that all the love, prayers, and positive energy sent our way have played in how astonishingly well things have gone up to this point.

With love and gratitude,
Kathryn

SEATTLE SIGHTS

Kathryn

August 18, 2014

Day +23: I am someone who likes change and I quickly tire of routine activities. Consequently, I'm getting restless with the day-to-day focus on my health and I need to find little ways that I can engage with the world as I recover. I like new projects, new people, and new places. Between work and family commitments, Dave and I feel like we have not thoroughly explored the city we live in. Since I am required to be no more than 30 minutes from Seattle Cancer Care Alliance for the next 3 months, I'm interested in suggestions that any of you may have for things to do around town. Due to diet restrictions, restaurants are out but we are open to all kinds of other ideas.

Meanwhile, Dave and I are trying to enjoy the very small pleasures in life and be good sports about not having any summer adventures, other than the one we're in the middle of (!) We are walking 3-4 miles daily and I do not appear to have graft versus host disease yet. Even if grubby campsites in other countries are out of the question a year from now, I do hope our life horizons will have expanded beyond a 30-minute radius of SCCA.

Thanks again for all the support during my hospitalization. We hope I won't be back there any time soon and will write here from time to time until I am discharged at Day 100.

All for now.

Love,
Kathryn

WEEK ONE AT HOME SUMMARY

Dave

August 19, 2014

Day +24: Being a caregiver is like a combination of two great memories from my past - dealing with a newborn infant, and shingling our cabin on Vashon.

Like dealing with infants it seems that every waking minute is occupied with details related to preparing food, cleaning up the mess afterwards, washing clothes, washing dishes, washing bodies, dealing with doctors appointments, going shopping to the drugstore, going shopping to the grocery store, taking deep breaths, rinsing and repeating all of those things again two or three more times in a day and then collapsing into a fitful sleep before getting up to do it all over again. Kathryn, of course, is not like an infant (even though I happen to think that she is just as adorable...). She is able to do at least half of all the activities involved but the amount of detail that goes into every step of every process is incredibly time consuming and requires both of our combined concentration.

How about some simple carrot and fennel soup for lunch? No problem. Just wash every carrot thoroughly before peeling, peel with a bleached-clean knife, rinse peeled carrot thoroughly again and then chop on the bleached-clean chopping board with another freshly bleach-cleaned knife, then add to the pot. Do the same with fennel, onion and other spices and ingredients, cook in "Magic Mineral Broth," blenderize the cooked soup into a delicious puree and keep in the fridge ready to use. Clean all the dirty utensils, chopping boards, pots and plates and then put them into the dishwasher. None of this is hard but it takes about three times as long as usual to prepare anything.

Kathryn's Hickman central IV line is a marvelous thing but takes a fair amount of attention. She gets a liter of 0.9% sodium chloride infused over 5 hours with varying amounts of magnesium, and potassium added depending on the results of her twice-weekly lab tests at SCCA. Hooking her up to this requires vigorous hand-washing, wearing gloves, swabbing the ends of the IV tubing with alcohol, flushing with saline, swabbing with more alcohol, flushing with heparin, connecting the liter of fluids to a portable infusion pump, making sure that we have supplies of alcohol swabs and spare batteries and clamps with us when she goes out wearing the rig, and repeating the swabbing and flushing process when the pump beeps to tell us it is done with the infusion.

Right now Kathryn is only taking 8 different varieties of pills. Some are taken singly, others twice a day, or four times a day, some on an empty stomach, others with food, some need to **not** be taken with others. Twice a week we withhold the morning dose of tacrolimus (the "Roman centurion" who is protecting Kathryn from the over-zealous new stem cells) until we get a blood level checked in the lab so we carry a backpack to SCCA filled with pill bottles and notepads to make adjustments as needed.

So our days are spent in these repeated and rather humdrum tasks where attention to detail is paramount. This is why it reminded me of the time (about fifteen years ago) when Lewis helped me to shingle our little cabin on Vashon. It was satisfying manual labor that required attention to lots of details of measurement and selection, with plumb lines, spirit levels and chalk lines, and cutting and pounding. He and I made lots of mistakes but by the time we were putting on the last few pieces right up in the peak of the gable end at the front we felt we had made all our mistakes, had learned from them, and had finally figured out how to do it well. In other words it was only by the time we were finished that we felt competent to do the job! And yet we may never have to shingle another building in our lives, and if we do it will be long enough in the future that we will no doubt have already forgotten how to avoid our mistakes and so will probably make them all over again! With all this immunosuppressed hyper-clean cooking, flushing and swabbing of IV lines, and setting up mobile infusion pumps I am managing to make an interesting variety of mistakes and so have had to redo some things several times. I feel as though I am getting better and more skilled at it the longer I do it so perhaps by the time I am really good at all of this I will no longer need to do it any more! I'd be fine with that.

So far, though, things are going well for Kathryn. Her various bodily discomforts are lessening and our only concern at the moment is that her liver function tests (a sensitive measure of the level of enzymes that her liver produces) have been rising over the last 3-4 tests. This may be due to having too high a level of tacrolimus or may be a side effect of another of the drugs (fluconazole) and so they are making adjustments and repeating the lab tests in a few days. If the liver enzymes keep rising then they will look for other causes. It is possible that this is an early sign of graft-versus-host (GVH) disease but they don't think so. Whatever they find we will adjust and roll with it. We were told today, by one of the senior SCCA physicians whom we trust and respect, that the longer a person goes without getting problems like infections or fevers or skin rashes or other problems then the less likely they are to get those problems. Yes, it is still most likely that GVHD will occur at some point but the longer it is before it declares itself to be a problem then the milder and more amenable it is likely to be to treatment. No guarantees, but everything is still looking pretty good.

So here's hoping for another quiet, humdrum, boring week of repetitive tasks, and uneventful walks in the woods.

PAINTING BY NUMBERS

Dave

August 28, 2014

Day +33.3... I was barely three years old when I discovered the joys of expressing myself in visual "art." My mom would sit me down at the kitchen table in the schoolhouse at Mahaar with a pencil or a crayon and a pile of scrap paper and away I would go. Birds were my preferred muse, apparently. My mom has described it vividly. I would grip the crayon firmly, press it down on the paper and draw a bird in one bold clockwise movement without lifting the crayon again: beak... head... back... tail... big round belly... neck... head... and back to the beak. I'd then lift up the crayon and add a dot for the eye, two spindly legs and maybe a squiggle for the wings. I would then proudly announce, "Bidd!" before starting on another. I was nothing if not prolific.

My mother clearly thought she had a genius on

her hands because she carefully preserved some of my earliest efforts for posterity. I saw them again for the first time in about 55 years when I found a faded brown envelope full of my bird drawings when clearing out the family house after my dad died last year. Picasso may have had his "Blue Period" but young David clearly had his "Bird Period!" Now that I have kids and grandkids of my own I see nothing particularly amazing about my own early drawings. I am much more impressed by the artwork that my own offspring have produced. But one thing that all of these childhood pictures have in common is their exuberance and creativity. You just give yourself a blank page, let your imagination wander and see where it takes you...

A few years later, when I was out of my "Bird Period" and into my "Monsters With Fierce Eyes And Large Teeth Period" one of my aunts thought that it was high time that I learned how to do "real art." I was given a very important looking ***Painting By Numbers*** present. It came in its own box, with real paintbrushes and a couple of dozen tiny plastic pots of paint with exotic names like "Burnt Sienna" and "Aquamarine." It also came with detailed instructions, which my mother made clear I **HAD** to follow! The picture itself, I remember, was a pastoral landscape scene: an idyllic English country cottage with fruit trees in the foreground, forests and mountains in the background. There wasn't a bird or a monster to be seen anywhere! Not one. Even worse, there were no blank pieces of paper or cardboard on which to smear the burnt sienna paint messily and exuberantly. No, no, no, the instructions were quite explicit. The lid of the box showed you what the finished picture was supposed to look like. Inside the box was a single rectangle of thick white card on which there was a black and white outline of the same pastoral scene. Each section of the picture was carefully separated from the neighboring sections with crisp, clean black lines and the area thus enclosed was given a number. It might be "11" or "17." There might be a dozen "17s" scattered across the page. I amused myself by counting to see which number appeared most often while my mom continued to give me her careful instructions. The little pots of paint were also numbered, you see? My job was to open pot "17," for example, dip my paintbrush into it ("and be careful not to be wasteful and apply too much paint, David") and then find all of the little squiggly-shaped sections on the picture that had a "17" in the middle of them. I should then carefully ("... very carefully, David, be sure you stay within the lines!") fill in that section of the picture with whatever color "17" was.

I thought it might be more fun to start in one corner of the picture and paint the first section with its color and then switch to the color of the adjacent section and proceed like this so that the painting emerged as if it was a multicolored flag being unfurled. But I was quickly told that this was **NOT** what to do! This was against the rules! This was wasteful! Every time you changed color you needed to use a new brush or wash the previous color out before you could use the new color. Ve-e-e-ery wasteful! Besides, if you were a careless little boy, careless enough to stray outside of the lines into a recently painted section... before it was dry... the new color could bleed into that other color creating some entirely **NEW** color that was **NOT** in the original painting! Can you not see what a complete disaster that would be...? It gives a person shivers of panic just to think about it... No, no, no, the correct way to proceed was to do all of the "17s" at once and then let them dry... thoroughly... before selecting a new color for an adjacent section. If "17" was a shade of purple, for example, it might be used on a section of a plum hanging off a fruit tree in the foreground, be part of the shadow of the cottage, a patch of heather on the distant hillside and finally be a section of the underbelly of a thunder cloud in the sky up above. You could only do a few colors on any given day provided they did not include adjacent sections. You could then come back a few days later to apply some new numbered colors to other sections when everything else was dry. In this way over the course of a tedious couple of weeks the pastoral scene gradually became less and less black and white and turned into a colored version that was only marginally more interesting. Did I mention that there were no birds or monsters to be found anywhere in the picture. None! Not even hiding behind the plum tree or lurking in the purple shadow of the cottage. And even if you had half a pot of "Burnt Sienna" left at the end (because you had been extremely careful about not overusing it, I might add) you were **NOT** allowed to add a flaming orange bird in the perfect "Aquamarine" blue sky or an orange snake with dripping fangs hanging down from the plum tree. No, no, no. That was against the rules. You follow the instructions, David. You pay attention to the numbers and you **stay within the lines...**

Right now, here on **Day +33** (although since I am writing this after 8am it is technically **Day +33.3** so we are officially through the first THIRD of the "100 days" that we have heard so much about) Kathryn and I feel trapped within that bland pastoral scene from my childhood years ago. Our conversations are very detailed and specific. Our life is being **Painted By Numbers:**

"What day is it today, 34?"

"No, tomorrow will be Day 34. We go to the clinic tomorrow. Remember to ask about going back on Bactrim now that we are beyond Day 30."

"What was the AST on Tuesday?"

"It was 105. Although that is technically higher than the 104 we got last Friday that is within the expected lab error. It is definitely not rising as fast as it was so maybe whatever was causing it is plateauing and not getting worse. Let's just wait to see what number we get next Friday."

"What was your last neutrophil count/magnesium level/hematocrit/platelet count...?"

"That was the nurse at SCCA. She says my Tacrolimus level was only 4 which is sub therapeutic so we need to increase my dose from 1.5mg twice a day to 2.0mg twice a day. I'm pretty sure we have capsules of 1mg and 0.5 mg strength in the dresser upstairs. Could you just go and double-check that we have the right dose in the Mediset starting tonight until we get my next Tacro level done?"

"How long has your saline infusion been running?"

"About three and a half hours."

"Okay, well there was 990mls in the bag when we got you hooked up this morning and it runs at 200mls an hour so you've got over an hour left before we need to disconnect you from that, clean and clear both your lines, and get your Micofungin hooked up..."

There will come a day when we can disregard the numbers, throw caution to the wind, and let as much "Burnt Sienna" as we like bleed recklessly into whatever neighboring color it is around! I am not suggesting that this will be anytime soon. I am not going to show the cosmos just how daring and reckless I can be by only washing and rinsing every **other** kale leaf from now on. That would be stupid. Right now we have no way to know which corners we could possibly cut so we will continue to color very carefully within the lines, follow all the instructions to the letter, and pay close attention to the numbers.

But one of these days in the not too distant future Kathryn Crawford will gambol out into the meadow of life again and gaze at orange birds flying in the blue skies up above...

Bring on **Day +34**

A UNIFYING THEORY

Dave

August 30, 2014

Day +35 Spoiler Alert: *Some of you may not find this journal entry to be entertaining or interesting at all. You may not care about understanding the medical and technical details of what is happening to Kathryn. If so, feel free to skip this and go and do something fun. There will be no sappy childhood reminiscences here, no tortured analogies. Just facts. Medical facts, laboratory values, clinical observations, signs and symptoms. I am writing this to meet a need of my own. It is important for me to try to process the ever-changing barrage of data and information that Kathryn and I are receiving. Writing it down and trying to explain it in language that is easy to understand helps me to make sense of it so that Kathryn and I can deal with what is likely to be ahead for us.*

Okay, now to call this entry "A Unifying Theory"

might seem a bit grandiose. I did not, however, say that it was "**THE** Unifying Theory." You know the one - the theory that attempts to reconcile Einstein's theory of relativity, quantum mechanics, string theory, and the meaning of life all at the same time. This has already been done, of course. Not by academic astrophysicists like Stephen Hawking or Neil deGrasse Tyson but by that futuristic visionary, Douglas Adams, in his comprehensive academic tome, ***The Hitchhiker's Guide to the Galaxy***. Adams explains that the big question about the ultimate meaning of life was posed to a massive intergalactic computer, which processed all the information in the universe since the beginning of time and came up with the answer, which it then gave to the assembled masses... I won't spoil it for you by giving you the answer here. The Hitchhiker's Guide to the Galaxy is well worth a read or re-read.

The problem that I have been struggling to make sense of is that the information about how Kathryn is doing so far is mixed. It is mostly good, for sure, but not all of the information fits together well and some of it could be bad. Here's the summary:

Kathryn is generally looking and feeling better each day. She has more energy, she can go for 4+ mile walks at a good clip, she is eating well, and her bodily functions are mostly behaving. Yes, she has some skin discoloration and itching and has problems getting to sleep and staying asleep and I am not minimizing any of those but in general she seems to me to be steadily improving. So all that seems **good**.

But her liver function tests are rising, and that seems **bad**. Now the liver does a whole host of important things for us but two important ones are clearing toxins out of the body and producing a yellow substance called bile, which helps us to absorb fat from our diet. That bile flows in tiny little tubes that join to make bigger tubes like the tributaries of a river until it flows to the gall bladder, down the bile duct and into your guts. Now if the flow of bile gets interrupted and backs up the person can turn yellow (doctors call that ***jaundice*** since jaune is the French word for yellow and it sounds wa-a-ay more important and serious and medical to use a foreign word to describe it). You can also tell that the bile is backing up by seeing two chemicals (bilirubin and alkaline phosphatase) rise in the blood. That is a common pattern if there is graft-versus-host-disease(GVHD) in the liver. But that is not what we are seeing with Kathryn. Instead it is her liver enzymes alanine amino transferase (ALT) and aspartate amino transferase (AST) that are rising. That can happen if anything is irritating or inflaming the liver cells. While this can happen with GVHD it is less common. It can certainly happen if the liver gets inflamed because of a viral infection (viral hepatitis) or could happen because of a chemical injury (from chemo-drugs, for example). For Kathryn the puzzling thing is that her AST and ALT were normal until Day +20, rose quickly until Day +27 and have been more or less stable and flat at a somewhat higher level (AST around 108 and ALT around 200) since then. If this was progressive GVHD or a viral infection we would expect Kathryn to feel worse, probably have a fever, and the rise would be much faster and more relentless).

Kathryn has no loss of appetite (anorexia), no pain in her belly, no diarrhea, and has never had any fever. All these are **good** and not what we'd expect if she had major GVHD developing or had a rip-roaring viral infection of the liver.

Her blood counts for red blood cells, white blood cells and platelets all began rising vigorously starting after Day +10 and rose steadily for the next ten days so that she has not ever needed any more red cell or platelet infusions since then. All that is **good** but they have plateaued since then and are "stuck" at a level that is reasonable but not as high as we would ultimately like or expect them to be, so that is a bit **bad**.

The bone marrow biopsy that she had last Tuesday at four weeks (actually it was on Day +31) was "unsatisfactory" in that it showed quite a bit of fibrous tissue still in the marrow and not as much evidence of healthy production of red and white cells and platelets as they would like, so that is kind of **bad**, although not unexpected in someone who had myelofibrosis before her transplant.

When they look at the blood samples they get from Kathryn under the microscope then can see some "nucleated red cells." Those are primitive red cells that are usually only found in the bone marrow. In a healthy state they stay in the marrow and the only cells that are released into the peripheral blood stream are mature little red donuts with no nuclei. So finding nucleated red blood cells in the peripheral blood is not what we want to see, so might be **bad**.

The senior doctor on our team for this month (the "Attending Physician") is a wonderful man called Fred Applebaum. He is a world expert in the field and has worked with many thousands of patients going through stem cell transplantation over the last three decades. He is also a really good listener, a great communicator, and a kind and thoughtful guy (a winning combination, for sure!). I could tell that he has been trying to reconcile all of these observations into one plausible and coherent story, too. Yesterday he offered us the following possible explanation:

The donated stem cells (the "Jersey girls") are doing great. They engrafted quickly which means that they found enough space among the fibrous tissue in Kathryn's bone marrow to "set up shop" and start producing red cells, white cells and platelets. From Day +10 through Day +20 those all rose steadily into a useful range so that Kathryn has not required transfusions and can walk 4+ miles a day without getting breathless or tired. The fact that they haven't risen higher, however, might mean that there just isn't enough room within Kathryn's bone marrow yet to keep increasing production by opening up more assembly lines. The "inadequate" bone marrow biopsy on Day +31 shows that there is still a fair amount of fibrous tissue in her marrow. Fibrous cells turn over very slowly and so it may be several more months before they get "cleaned out" by the effects of the conditioning chemotherapy and destruction by the new stem cells.

In the meantime those vigorous new stem cells from Jersey are looking to find alternative accommodation outside of the bone marrow in which to make their new blood cells. The fancy medical Latin term for this is "extramedullary hematopoiesis." One of the most favored places where they like to do this is in the liver. After all, it is a big soft organ with a great blood supply and room to expand inside your belly. So it is possible that a few million stem cells are "muscling their way" into the liver and pushing some of the liver cells out of their way in the process. Those neighboring liver cells may be getting a bit irritated by this and are releasing enzymes (ALT and AST) into the bloodstream to "voice their complaint." Those liver function tests were in the normal range until Day +20, rose sharply between Day +20 and +27 but appear to be leveling off or rising much more slowly since then. This is all more compatible with extramedullary hematopoiesis than with liver GVHD or a viral infection of the liver. While both of those latter things are still possible they seem less likely with what we are seeing.

Dr. Applebaum was cautious about all of this. It is just a theory that fits well with all of the data we have. The only way to be sure that this unifying theory is correct would be to stick a big needle into Kathryn's liver and look at all of the cells under a microscope to see what they are doing. That is a somewhat painful and dangerous procedure and so for now he suggested that we simply continue to observe how Kathryn does over the next several weeks. If the "hepatic extramedullary hematopoiesis" theory is correct then the AST and ALT may stay up for several months. But over those same months we may see Kathryn's blood counts gradually rise further as the fibrous tissue gets cleaned out of her marrow leaving more room for additional "factory production lines" to be set up there, since the bone marrow is their preferred location.

This may all be wishful thinking on my part but I find this Unifying Theory very reasonable and quite reassuring. There are plenty of other new things that may well show up and cause problems for us but for now we will continue to track Kathryn's energy level, symptoms, temperature, skin appearance, appetite, lab values, and hope for the best.

DARTH VADER IN A HANDBAG

Dave

September 1, 2014

Day +37: Today is Labor Day. The last hurrah of summer. Kathryn's extended family will be congregating on Vashon Island. Our kids and grandkids are getting excited about the new school year that is about to start. Signs of impending autumn are in the air. My mom used to say that summer was coming to an end when the last blooms of Rose Bay could be seen on the verges and woodlands around Scotland. Rose Bay Willow Herb (also known as Fireweed) is also a plentiful wild flower/weed in the Pacific Northwest but seems to come and go in the middle of the summer here rather than signaling the approach of autumn. The signs that Kathryn and I most often look for in the waning days of summer are that blackberries are getting overripe, some leaves start turning color, spider webs appear overnight almost every single day, and flying ants flap confusedly around the porch light at night time.

This end of summer has felt distinctly different for us this year, of course. Kathryn is usually a vigorous and determined blackberry picker. Like so many things in her life she has developed a very effective system for blackberry collection. We have some great patches near the family cabin on Vashon, on the steep hill on our driveway, and along the nearby roadside. For me, one of Kathryn's most "fetching" outfits is to see her wearing a long-sleeved flannel shirt (to ward off bramble thorns), jeans tucked into rubber boots (to avoid nettle stings on the ankles) and a battered straw hat (to get some shade from the sun) and wearing her milk-carton-and-pantyhose-blackberry-collector over her head. Kathryn has gathered up some plastic one-gallon milk cartons over the years, washed and rinsed them and cut the top off while leaving the plastic handle intact. She then attaches old pantyhose (often with spots of nail polish on them where rips and holes have been repaired before they became too battered for daily use on her legs) to the milk carton handle so that a person can drape this over their head and around their neck. This means the milk carton is held at about chest height leaving both arms free for blackberry picking. The picked blackberries can be deposited in the milk carton. You know it is getting too full when the carton drops down to waist level and the pantyhose is cutting into the back of your neck.

As with so many other things in life the juiciest blackberries are always just out of reach hovering over a patch of nettles or far above the outstretched arms. But to an undaunted Kathryn most of these delicacies eventually give up their wares by judicious placement of planks of wood and ladders out into the bramble patch. Seeing Kathryn stretched out precariously high above the nettles and briars with her fingers straining out in front of her and a steely look in her eye is one of my most enduring memories of summertime. We usually pick several pounds - enough to make blackberry cobbler, blackberry crumble (using my mom's recipe where the topping is essentially thick chunks of butter shortbread), blackberry jam (both regular and freezer jam) and sometimes bramble jelly (where bags of cooked blackberries are strained through muslin bags so that the seeds and pulp are kept back and only the purple nectar gets through to be turned into sticky tastiness). We have missed out on all of those activities this year (the bramble scratches, the nettle stings, the aching backs, as well as the marvelous smells, tastes and sights of pots and 9 by 13 glass Pyrex dishes brimming with purple jewels covering the table and other kitchen surfaces). But there will be more blackberry-picking summers to come...

So what have you all been up to on this Labor Day? I hope you have had fun with friends and family getting sunburn and mosquito bites while waterskiing, fishing, jumping off the dock or grilling overcooked and charred burgers on the deck, all washed down with cold beer or Margaritas. This year I did something a bit different - I went for a walk with Darth Vader in a handbag. Actually Kathryn came too, which made it even more fun. One of the long lists of irritations and inconveniences that Kathryn has to suffer right now is that her skin is under assault in every crack and crevice of her body. It burns, chafes and itches like the devil, especially on places where there is extra pressure on it. But she also needs to get daily exercise and needs to get tanked up with intravenous fluids and electrolytes. As I mentioned in a previous journal entry we have a portable infusion pump and a little backpack that holds the pump, the liter bag of fluids and the tubing to connect this to her central Hickman IV line. Lugging this around causes the skin on Kathryn's shoulder to itch and get angry and discolored so we have concocted a system whereby we pull out an additional few feet of plastic tubing so that I can walk beside her and hold the little backpack containing the saline bag and the pump as it slowly dispenses its liter of precious fluids over five hours. This gives Kathryn a few blessed minutes of relative freedom but it adds a level of complexity to our walks through Discovery Park because I need to make sure there is enough slack in the tubing so that Kathryn does not get tugged on when she speeds up or slows down or dives off into one side of the path or other in search of something of interest. She already feels that she is on a short enough leash in her life these days as it is, without that!

But this also adds a new level of excitement to my walks because it feels as though I am carrying Darth Vader in a handbag. The infusion pump makes a rather loud, long, sucking sound every few seconds that reminds me of the sound that Darth Vader makes inside that sinister black mask of his in the Star War movies. Now I know what you're thinking. "Good grief, how unutterably dull has Dave's life become that he has to manufacture an elaborate fantasy world around him to spice it up!" But hang on a minute. You don't think that I go on our walk imagining that there are Imperial Storm Troopers firing lasers at us through the woods, do you? I'm not **that** juvenile. That would be ridiculous. There is no way that Storm Troopers would be stupid enough to fire lasers at us if they knew that I was carrying Darth Vader in my handbag. Have some common sense! Even if they managed to "take out" Kathryn and me, if they killed DV in the process they would be in bi-i-i-ig trouble with the Emperor (and the lightning bolts that he can fire from his wizened and gnarly old hands). And I am not spending my time looking up above to see if Ewoks are about to dump rocks on our heads from the branches above. That would be even more ridiculous! The Ewoks clearly know that we are "good guys" because of that "Rebel Alliance" vibe we exude as we carefully make our way through the more treacherous patches of woods in Discovery Park...

No, the real danger that we face is from exuberant dogs and distracted teenagers who go careening along the paths while plugged into their iPods... the teenagers, that is. I have yet to see a dog wearing ear buds and an iPod, although living in Seattle I wouldn't be that surprised if I did. However, most dogs seem to be able to grin from ear to ear with happiness without any extra technology strapped to their heads. But if either of those creatures (teenagers or dogs) rushed between Kathryn and me on our walk and ripped out the plastic tubing that would be really **BAD**, so it adds some spice to the walk and keeps me on my toes making sure we avoid disaster.

Back at home our domestic life gets a little more complicated every day as more drugs are added to

Kathryn's pile. Our trashcan also looks a bit different these days filled with non-hazardous medical plastic packing material. The syringes and needles and hazardous stuff fill up separate containers that get mailed back to the company to get disposed of safely. Our fridge is full of bags of saline and magnesium. She is also now being given anti fungal prophylaxis using a drug called Micofungin that is dispensed in little balls that look like hand grenades and dispense their contents through the central line over the course of an hour. It looks like something you might see in a Star Wars movie.

Enough of the fantasy! We have clinic at SCCA again tomorrow so we will get a big dose of reality and will see where the numbers will take us from there.

CHANGING SEASONS

Kathryn

September 5, 2014

As summer drifts into autumn, Dave and I feel like we are in a period of transition and are moving into a new phase of my treatment process. I find myself reflecting on my year of health challenges. In February I learned that I had a life-threatening illness, myelofibrosis, and that I had two treatment options. One was palliative care until I died, and the other was a stem cell transplant, if a donor could be found. I considered both options with care.

If I chose palliative care, my symptoms would steadily worsen and I might live a couple of years. If I had a transplant, it would be a long and risky process but it might extend my life, possibly by many years. There was also a chance that I'd live a few miserable months and die sooner than if I had chosen palliative care. Each option would involve a lot of misery but, since there was some hope embedded in the transplant path, that's what I decided to do.

I am now 41 days post transplant. The treatment requires a commitment to live within 30 minutes of SCCA for four months and to have a dedicated caregiver for all that time. I am incredibly lucky to have a very devoted, smart, and good-humored caregiver in my dear husband. His role is just about as challenging and time consuming as mine, and it's clear to both of us now why they require caregivers for as long as they do.

As fall approaches, Dave and I are adjusting to the reality of the very long and uncertain treatment path ahead. We have been told that the first 100 days post-transplant always feel like a roller coaster and that most people don't start feeling close to some kind of normal for about a year.

Since Dave is right by my side through all of this, it really feels like a team effort. I've caught myself referring to "our" appointments. I guess that makes sense since I am still not driving so he attends all of them with me. We now have appointments 4 days/week. I'm not sure I would survive this without him; I certainly wouldn't be doing as well as I am.

As we've written previously, our biggest worry now is how bad my graft-versus-host-disease (GVHD) will be, the new cells recognizing my body as foreign and attacking healthy organs cause it. In these early days, it most commonly affects the skin, the gut, and the liver. I was told I had an 80% chance of getting it and I already have the skin form and probably have it in my mouth. What that means for me is that my upper body is incredibly itchy and my mouth is so dry that food doesn't taste great and my lips feel tight. I would give a lot for a few hours of physical comfort.

My liver enzymes have been rising so the team is trying to determine whether or not I also have it in my liver. The standard treatment for GVHD is massive doses of prednisone. As some of you will know, prednisone is an incredibly powerful and effective steroid drug with some nasty side effects. They include bone loss, muscle wasting, insomnia, mood swings, development of diabetes, and a puffy face. Needless to say, if I develop diabetes I will be in excellent hands, since Dave is a diabetes specialist. For any of you medical readers, until it's clear whether or not I have liver GVHD, they are trying an interesting treatment for my skin called PUVA. (If I have it in my liver I have to go straight to prednisone.) The abbreviation stands for psoralen ultraviolet A, and the idea is to avoid the prednisone if possible. The treatment involves me taking a drug, oxsoralen, 90 minutes before stripping naked and getting into a tanning booth for 58-65 seconds. The nurse operator was pleased that I'd never seen a tanning booth before. However, I had to confess that as a teen I covered refrigerator boxes in tin foil and laid under them with baby oil on to maximize my tan.

Regarding medications, a new doctor this week commented on how few medications I am on! Some of you have seen the pictures of my medications on this site and, for someone who was on one medication before my transplant, I have not been thanking my lucky stars for how few I am on now. The doctor's comment changed my perspective and I am now appropriately grateful. Adjusting my perspective on many things has been a major feature of this journey. I have been told more than once that this process will age me 10 years in one. Hard to know what that really means but I will do all I can to maximize my function even if I appear 10 years older next summer. I am being monitored very carefully and I am sure that the excellent SCCA providers do not have me on a single drug that I don't really need.

Dave and I know that we need to plan on some dark days ahead. Dave has said this feels like a really slow, bad movie but we have to sit through it until the end. Our hope is that eventually there will be a pretty happy ending but we are not offered any guarantees. It may be a really long bad movie with a lousy ending. This is the aspect of our current experience that is the hardest to live with day to day. We really feel like we could do ANYTHING for a year if we knew it was going to get us to a better place. In this situation, we must do all we can to maximize chances of things going well and accept that we do not control the most important factors related to GVHD.

We will write here from time to time and apologize for the fact that our posts will not always be cheery. When people have asked what they can do for us, the most important thing is keeping it real. For me, the only way through difficulty and grief is to allow myself to feel it all and know that if I do I will come out the other side. I sometimes feel like one of those weighted dolls that you push over and they bounce back up. With each new blow, I feel determined to try to keep coming back up.

Dave's love and good humor buoy my spirits on a daily basis and so does the love I feel from all of you. Although we may never really feel "out of the woods," we do hope that I feel increasingly better as I get to the six-month mark and that we feel sort of back to some kind of normal life by a year. It would be wonderful indeed if I was out picking berries on Vashon by the time they are ripe next year.

I hope all of you are finding time to savor these waning days of summer.

Thanks for all the love and encouragement.

Kathryn

A BAD, SLOW MOVIE WITH A CONVOLUTED PLOT

Dave

September 12, 2014

Day +51: As we move into the second half of the first hundred days since Kathryn's stem cell transplant I must confess that I am feeling a bit weary. Obviously, "100 days" is a somewhat random or arbitrary number and there is much variation in what underlying diseases different people have, how good their general health is before they start, how good their "donor match" is, and many other factors involved. Because of that, how well each person does is enormously variable. And yet having done thousands of stem cell transplants for the past few decades, SCCA has come to the conclusion that no matter how all these differences stack up for different individuals going through the process you can be assured that you need to have a full time caregiver for the first 100 days and that during that time you can expect a LOT of different problems to show up and setbacks to face. We are living through all of that right now.

Kathryn has mentioned that I have often referred to what we are going through as like being forced to sit through a really slow, bad movie. That is true. I have. So as I have done in the past, what I try to do for myself (and for anyone who cares to read these journal entries) is to try to challenge myself about how I am feeling and examine those feelings in a little more detail. Is that a reasonable analogy? What are the attributes of a movie that make me dislike it and are those the things that are going on for us right now?

For me a movie is bad if:

There are no likable characters in it. Well that's not the problem here! I love the protagonist in this story. She is plucky, courageous, good humored, complex, layered, and with the right mixture of strengths and vulnerabilities that make you (the reader or viewer) want to root for her. A whole lot of the other characters whom we have met as the story unfolds are likable, too. Many of the doctors and nurses and other staff whom we have met in the hospital and in the various clinics before and after the hospital stay have been interesting and entertaining to differing degrees.

There are too many characters in it. This is certainly becoming part of the problem for me. Every month we need to get used to a different "attending (or senior academic) physician" plus a new "mid-level" (either a Physicians Assistant [PA] or an Advanced Registered Nurse Practitioner [ARNP]) along with other changes when anyone goes on vacation. We have also been sent to various extra appointments, which brings in new characters to deal with. We had a very unsatisfactory appointment with gastroenterology where Kathryn first had to tell her story to a foreign research fellow who claimed to have read through Kathryn's chart and then proceeded to ask asinine questions that made it clear that he hadn't. He then left us twiddling our thumbs for over half an hour before the senior gastroenterologist came back in with the research fellow. This guy was a caricature of an aloof academic physician who made it clear that he didn't think Kathryn's case was all that interesting or challenging, made a few vague suggestions for other tests he could do but ended up shrugging his shoulders and saying we should probably just wait and see how things developed over the next few weeks before deciding... He and his sidekick were two eminently forgettable characters!

The plot is too long. That is rarely a problem for me with a movie if I find the story very compelling. ***"Braveheart"*** was over three hours long and the ***"Lord of the Rings"*** trilogy is about ten hours long and for me all of those movies were too short! No, I knew that the "movie" we are now in the middle of would be long and I have been braced for that aspect, so that is not what is making it a "bad movie" for me.

The plot is boring and predictable. Again, that is NOT the problem with this movie! Some aspects of our day-to-day chores are certainly boring and repetitive but the overall plot is extremely unpredictable and the variety of plot twists is certainly not boring.

The plot is too convoluted and confusing. For me this CAN be a problem but not always. I can enjoy a really convoluted and confusing plot if it has a really clever and satisfactory ending! One of my favorite movies is ***"The Usual Suspects"*** (1995 starring Kevin Spacey and several other great actors). It has a very convoluted and confusing plot but a jaw-droppingly clever ending. On the other hand the movie ***"Mulholland Drive"*** (2001 starring Naomi Watts) was confusing from start to finish and, for me, the biggest waste of three hours I have endured in quite some time (understanding, of course, that people are all very different in what they like and don't like in movies! For all I know Mulholland Drive might be on your top ten favorite movies of all time!)

It has a really bad ending. This of course is the nub of the issue for me with the "movie" that Kathryn and I find ourselves in right now. We have no way of knowing how long the movie will last and there are no guarantees that the ending will be "good." In fact we have been warned several times that we should be very flexible in what our definition of "good" or "acceptable" might be as the plot unfolds. Not only that but we are not allowed to walk out in the middle of this movie and we can't fast-forward to see what the ending is like before deciding if it is worth sticking it out. We can't replay old scenes a few more times to try to understand them better, either. We just have to try to stay optimistic and hope that the ending won't be "too bad."

I am going to resist stretching the movie metaphor too far. I won't liken Kathryn to Frodo Baggins in the Lord of the Rings movies. That would make me Samwise Gamgee, her affable, good-natured, slightly simple-minded-but optimistic sidekick. That doesn't work on so-o-o-o-o many levels. However, I am struck that what Kathryn and I are in the middle of is indeed a long, epic, and uncertain journey in which the dangers and miseries that we have to face keep changing as we travel along. We have left behind our worries about whether there was any viable treatment option at all, whether we would find a suitable donor, whether Kathryn would be fit enough to survive myeloablative conditioning drugs, the anxiety about whether or not engraftment would happen, when it would happen, whether or not Kathryn would get infections and fevers and die before the graft "kicked in." We got to "Rivendell" (the transplant unit at 7NE) and were able to survive all that and emerge from it in better shape with a better chance of survival and the ability to continue on our journey.

The biggest "demon" that we need to wrestle with at this point is the GVHD-monster. We were told that there was an 80% chance of meeting it at some point on the journey but just how big, bad, and nasty he/she/it would be was, of course, uncertain... Well, GVHD is now well and truly upon us but it is still unclear how hard to deal with it will be.

[Spoiler Alert - some of you might find this to be a tedious medical sidebar:

They used to categorize graft-versus-host disease (GVHD) into three kinds depending on when it shows up and how it manifests itself. 1. ***Hyperacute*** *can come on within days of getting the stem cell transplant and indicates that the new cells really don't like where they find themselves and so vigorously attack the recipient's body. This can be very hard to treat, can kill you, and usually has a bad prognosis. Well, we dodged that bullet. Kathryn didn't get that. 2.* ***Acute*** *can come on anytime in the first 100 days and usually affects the skin, liver or guts with dramatic symptoms (rash, jaundice,* *severe diarrhea, among other things). It is often sudden and severe in how it makes its appearance. Again, Kathryn hasn't really developed anything that is like that. 3.* **Chronic**, *which typically comes on after 100 days and can affect any organ in your body. The manifestations can be a lot slower to make themselves clear. Nowadays that thinking is changing since these three categories (particularly Acute and Chronic) can overlap a lot.* ***...end of medical sidebar]***

Kathryn is showing signs and symptoms that could be GVHD within the first 100 days but the onset seems (so far at least) to be slow and gradual. She had some skin rash that was itchy. A skin biopsy showed some signs that were compatible with chronic GVHD and others that were more like "busulfan damage" from hospital chemotherapy, still other features were "equivocal" (which means that the pathologist looking at it under the microscope couldn't be sure what it was or what was causing it). She has some slowly rising liver function tests but they were NOT of the pattern typical of "Acute liver GVHD."

Kathryn's wise and Gandalf-like attending physician from last month, Fred Applebaum, suggested that since it wasn't entirely clear what was causing the rash we might try "Potentiated (or Psoralen-modified) Ultra Violet A" treatment, or PUVA. This might improve the rash without the need for very high dose prednisone treatment. As Kathryn has described, she started this about two weeks ago and it certainly seems to be helping. The rash is NOT getting worse and is NOT itchy anymore (Yay, a small victory, we hope). But our new, younger attending physician (who is nice and seems sharp and decisive) cut through the waffle from the unhelpful gastroenterology characters and said it is most likely that the skin and the rising LFTs are indeed a slow, grumbling manifestation of GVHD and so, in addition to the PUVA, we should try a moderate dose of prednisone for a week and see how Kathryn responds (in terms of how she feels overall, what happens to the skin rash and what happens to her liver function tests). We will see this new attending again tomorrow after a week of prednisone in addition to the PUVA and so we should have more information and some new decisions to make tomorrow.

Just for fun:

I went on Google and Bing and searched for "Top Ten Most Boring Movies." As you might imagine the lists that people came up with are very different. Most of them come from blogs written by opinionated "guys" who are particularly down on slow sappy "chick flick" movies. I am pleased to say that many of the movies on most of these lists were ones that I had not seen myself and so now probably won't. But one movie that did appear on several lists and which I have seen and did NOT like, was ***"The English Patient."*** The reviewer described it as follows:

The mind-numbingly dull story of a Hungarian mapmaker and his dying memories of the romance that tragically alters his life. Burned horribly in a fiery plane crash while crossing the Sahara Desert during WWII, he is tended to by a Canadian nurse with ghosts of her own...

Ouch!

And so the plot of our bad, slow movie continues to get more convoluted. Throughout all of this I need to keep reminding myself (as the seasoned staff at the SCCA clinic keep telling us) that Kathryn is "doing great" from their point of view. She has more energy and is having way fewer problems and complications than they often see at this stage... all of which makes them think that the "ending" to this movie should be really quite good. But none of us will know for sure for many, many more months. We just need to go get another large tub of popcorn from the concession stand and settle in for the next part of the adventure. Rivendell may be behind us but whether we are headed into the "Mines of Moria" (a ***"Lord of the Rings"*** reference) or "The Fire Swamp" (a reference to one of my all time favorite movies, ***"The Princess Bride"***) is unclear. Let's hope we don't have to climb up "The Cliffs of Insanity" before we get to ride off into the sunset...

COMPLICATED BIRTHDAY EMOTIONS

Dave

September 18, 2014

Day +54: Today is my 61st birthday so I am entitled to some maudlin' reflections. It was a year ago right now that Kathryn and I were flying back from Minneapolis after visiting Roderick and his family in Saint Paul and then seeing Dr. Teferri (world expert in myeloproliferative disease) at the Mayo Clinic. He gave us "good news" about why we should not worry about Kathryn's dropping blood counts. It was just a random blip, he said, and we could expect her to stay well with no changes for years and years. We were hugely relieved. And yet three months later we discovered that he was dead wrong about that, Kath had myelofibrosis, and nine months after that is where we are right now.

One year on, just last night, Kathryn burst into tears at dinner, shook with frustration, and sadness, and said that she didn't want all this for me and that I deserved better.

I beg to differ.

Kathryn Crawford is the best "gift," or "present" I have ever been given and that feeling keeps growing stronger and better and more true as the years go on. I couldn't find anyone out there in the world who comes **close** to being as good as she is, let alone better. She is the most interesting person I have ever found to talk to, the most fun person to travel with, stay at home with, go to bed with, discuss the troubles of the world with, make plans and dreams with, or ponder eternal questions with.

Obviously nothing about what we are going through is Kathryn's fault and while I wouldn't wish what we are going through on anyone, in many ways this, in itself, is another gift. Most couples don't get to go through adversity like this ever, or maybe only at the end of their lives, and we are a long way from that point. One of my favorite lines from one of my favorite Tom Waits songs (*Small Change, from* 1976) is where he is describing tragedy and adversity in a really seedy neighborhood of the city. He refuses to accept pity about the situation and snarls defiantly:

"Nah, the dreams ain't broken, down here,
They're just walking with a limp!"

That describes our situation very well. We both need to have patience and grit to get through this and Kathryn has plenty of both.

Among the many qualities and attributes that Kathryn has are her fierce honesty and her brilliantly clear communication. She can sweep aside unhelpful platitudes and wishy-washy dithering suggestions. She tackles the complexity of our current situation with a structure, logic, and clarity of thought that is breathtaking to watch and a delight to share in and support. These intense, complex, tedious days of figuring out drug doses, lab values, and appointment times are truly a gift to me. Being around Kathryn for hours and hours is never boring and is full of richness and pleasure for me. Neither your dreams nor your spirit are broken, here, Kathryn. Frankly, they're not even walking with a limp. I can barely keep up...

Kathryn has described the feeling of dread that she has whenever we go to the lab or the clinic because more often than not the news is bad, not good. She is getting used to dealing with repeated body blows. She has said that it is like being one of those inflatable toys with the weighted, rounded bottom that get punched flat to the ground but keep on coming back up again for more punishment. That's a nice analogy except that Kathryn is way cuter, has a nicer shape, a more interesting personality, and a bigger variety of moves than those punch bag dolls.

When we were at the clinic on Tuesday the latest "body blow" was that Kathryn's liver function tests have gotten worse, not better, since she was started on low dose prednisone last week. The smart, optimistic doctor was neither surprised nor disheartened. She said that we simply need to increase from a "wimpy" dose to a "real" (a.k.a. **bigger**) dose. I could tell that this was the last thing Kathryn wanted to hear but her response was typically "Kathronian." She said:

"Okay, so it is big doses of steroids over long

periods of time that can cause weak muscles and bone thinning, right? So what can I start doing **right now** to minimize those problems...?"

As soon as we got home from the clinic she insisted that we go out for our four mile walk through Discovery Park but when we got to the long flight of stairs (111 in total) that branch off to the left she said that we should go up and down them four or five times before continuing on the trail to give her buttocks and thighs a better work out to stave off prednisone-induced muscle wasting. So that's what we did and we will incorporate that into our new daily routine from now on...

I love that you face your demons head on, Kathryn. I love that you express your fears and frustrations and sadness with such honesty and candor. I am honored that you let me in to share all of this with you. I am not sure that I truly deserve the gift of Kathryn Crawford in my life but I savor every second that I get.

On this day of my birth the land of my birth is taking a historical vote on whether it should break away from England and become an independent nation. It is a complex issue that Kathryn and I have discussed during our recent walks and car trips. But last night we shared some laughs by watching a couple of Scottish stand up comedians skewering and dissecting the hypocrisy and stupidity of some of the politicians involved and the issues and arguments that they use to justify their own position. For any of you interested check out ***Kevin Bridges*** on YouTube.

Although I have tried to keep up with some of the arguments that are being made for and against Scottish independence I find it hard to decide, having lived in the

USA and away from Scotland for over 30 years, now. Recently I checked in with some of my friends and family who still live in Scotland to get their take. I particularly trust the opinion of Dave Godden. Dave and I have been best friends since we met in our first year at Edinburgh University back in 1971! Dave was an exceptionally good doctor and researcher (recently retired) and has had more than his own share of personal health adversity to deal with during his life. Yet through all of it he has remained one of the wittiest, most good-humored and upbeat people I have ever known. He commented that as the day for the vote has gotten closer and closer the stridor and vitriol of some people on either side of the debate has risen to unpleasant proportions. He gave me a great quote that summed up the situation perfectly. At the risk of offending some of you I will repeat it here, since I think it so perfectly captures irreverent Scottish humor!

"Having a political opinion is like having a big willie (Scottish slang term for a penis) - you can be quite proud of it and even share it with close friends, but you shouldn't go waving it about in public and you certainly shouldn't stick it down other people's throats!"

I am left with the feeling that no matter what the outcome of the vote on Scottish Independence, the nation will continue to thrive and grow because of the indomitable spirit and good humor of the people who live there.

I feel the same about the complex and confusing situation that Kathryn and I are in right now. We will have plenty to cry about but will find much to laugh about, too, as we continue this journey. We are learning so much about many things, including each other, along the way. I think it is making us wiser, stronger, and more humble and thoughtful travelers as we go along. I am very optimistic about where we will be and what our life and dreams will look like in the years ahead.

"BODY BLOWS" UPDATE - MORE COMPLEXITY

Dave

September 25, 2014

Day +61... *Spoiler Alert*: *This entry will be mostly technical/ medical detail that will not be of interest to all. Some of what I chronicle here may also seem like bad news or steps backwards to some of you but I honestly don't think it is either.*

What's going on with the liver? Kathryn's liver function tests (LFTs) continue to rise slowly (the AST and ALT but not the bilirubin or Alkaline Phosphatase). Her liver ultrasound showed a slightly enlarged liver and a small amount of fluid in the abdomen, but no obstruction and no fatty liver. The screening tests for liver viruses were all negative. The conclusion from all of that by the gastroenterologist is that this is most likely slowly progressive chronic GVHD of the liver (he was so convinced of this that he did not think it was necessary to stick a needle into Kathryn's liver to confirm his view with a biopsy). Kath was started on prednisone 0.5mg/kg/day **(moderate dose)** on Day +45. The LFTs were unchanged a week later and so the dose was increased to 1.0mg/kg/day **(big dose)** on Day +52. The LFTs are still unchanged to my eye (and I graphed them out to be sure) but the academic GI doc thinks that they may be plateauing and that we should give it all more time. We have several options at this point. We could increase the prednisone dose to 2.0mg/kg/day **(VERY big dose)**, or switch from tacrolimus to a different drug called **sirolimus** that might work better along with prednisone to suppress the GVHD and might allow us to get control at a lower prednisone dose. The GI doc wants to stick to the moderate dose of prednisone for now but also to try another newish approach by giving Kathryn **Beclomethasone-In-Corn-Oil** to take by mouth. They mostly use this to treat GVHD of the stomach and intestines. It is a steroid that is not absorbed much and so it is acts on the gut lining (similar to using a steroid cream on the skin). It is, however, taken up by the liver and as it passes through the liver it can cause some beneficial local effects there, too. Might help, won't hurt, so we start that today (half a teaspoon of oil four times a day).

Are there other implications of using this approach? Anyone who is immunosuppressed like Kathryn is at increased risk of developing infections from bacteria, fungi, or viruses and so she has been on prophylactic medicines to fend off all three categories of "bugs" since before they gave her the conditioning chemotherapy. Because adding high dose prednisone increases those risks then the prophylactic meds need to be adjusted. The antibacterial prophylaxis remains the same. Trimethoprim-Sulfamethoxazole ("Bactrim") taken two days a week remains the tried and true most effective thing they have (in the absence of having a specific bacterium to fight). The antifungal agent that Kathryn is taking (Micofungin) is a good one but they have doubled the dose from 50mg to 100mg. This is the drug that comes in the little "hand-grenades" that self-deflate over an hour and is given once a day as an infusion into Kathryn's central intravenous Hickman line. The new "grenades" are the same size as the old ones so we do not notice any practical difference. Presumably the "goo" inside them is more concentrated. For antiviral prophylaxis she had been on acyclovir but when the prednisone dose was increased to 1mg/kg/day last week they they changed this to the more powerful **valacyclovir**. That was not a big change - just a different size and color of pill taken twice a day. So far so good until...

Have there been other new wrinkles? We have known all along that Kathryn has been infected in the past by a virus called cytomegalovirus (or CMV). Many people, including a lot of you, will have encountered this virus at some time in your past when you had a particularly bad "head-cold" or "chest-cold" or "flu." We fight it off, develop antibodies to it so that the infection gets cured but the virus hangs around and stays dormant in our bodies for years and years afterwards. When a person gets their immune system wiped out and gets a new immune system from someone who has never been exposed to CMV (which is the case with Kathryn), and the person is then put on hefty doses of immunosuppressives, including steroids like prednisone, then there is a fairly high risk that CMV will "wake up" and cause mischief. The transplant team has been looking out for this. Kathryn has had lab tests at least once a week ever since her conditioning chemotherapy looking for signs that CMV might be about to cause problems. We found out at her clinic appointment yesterday that this day is now here and so even valacyclovir is not strong enough to fight off the CMV. Instead she has been started on **gancyclovir** (Doesn't that one even **sound** tougher, like it is part of a gang?) Unfortunately, gancyclovir needs to be given as yet another intravenous infusion through the Hickman line. It will be given twice a day (in more little self-deflating "hand-grenades") for a week and then once a day for another two weeks. The CMV activity will be watched carefully by lab tests during this time. Also, gancyclovir is considered "toxic" or hazardous in the same way that heavy duty chemo drugs like busulfan are and so I need to take extra precautions in handling it and in disposing of the little empty "grenades." We now have an even more colorful array of trash bags and "Sharps" containers decorating the upper floor of our house where we have our "medical station!"

So for those of you keeping tally at home or those who are using Kathryn's journey as an easy way to study for your Internal Medicine Board Recertification exams (!) here is the **Treatment Summary** (excluding innocuous minerals and vitamins):

- 4 daily infusions through the central IV line (saline and magnesium over 4 hours, gancyclovir twice (1 hour each time) and Micofungin once (over 1 hour).

- Tacrolimus 2mg twice a day
- 50 mg of Prednisone once a day
- Beclomethasone suspension four times a day
- Ursadiol 600mg three times a day
- Bactrim two days a week
- plus combinations of drugs to help with nausea, sleep, itch and pain that Kathryn takes very sparingly along with a drawerful of creams, ointments and potions to slather on her skin or other places or to gargle and swish with as needed...)

So how do things feel overall here on Day +61? Kathryn will write separately about how she is feeling at this stage. For me, keeping track of all of these drugs and infusions and the supplies that go with them along with preparing healthy food safely, staying tuned in to how Kathryn is feeling, and getting daily exercise along with her is a full time job. The complexity and every-changing nature of the treatment is both intellectually and emotionally exhausting. I am more than ready to collapse in bed by 7-8pm most nights. But as I step back and see the big picture of the path we are on I really feel quite optimistic. Kathryn got no hyperacute GVHD and no real acute GVHD either. Our transplant team says that the CMV issue is another common occurrence and one that they seem confident can be dealt with. Like 80+% of people in her situation Kathryn is having to deal with some chronic GVHD. Although this has shown up at an earlier stage than it often does, this in itself does **not** have bad long-term prognostic implications (we have asked several of our experts about this specifically and got the same definitive answer from each of them). In fact at this stage the chronic GVHD is not behaving in an "aggressive" manner. Almost all of the skin itching, rash, and discoloration have gone or are improving. She is eating well, exercising well, is good-humored (at least most of the time!), and is taking everything in her stride. We really enjoy each other's company, find lots and lots of things to reflect on and discuss, and we check in with each other whenever things seems too overwhelming for either of us.

We knew before we started down this path that this is not for the faint hearted. There are no shortcuts to recovery and no one gets through it without several "setbacks" or "complications" along the way. We are not in an easy patch, right now, but it is totally manageable. Deep breaths...

INVOLUNTARY COMPLEXITY

Kathryn

September 28, 2014

As my treatment regimen seems to become ever more complicated, I find myself thinking back to the early 90's when I joined a small group of people on Vashon exploring concepts related to trying to live simply, the "voluntary simplicity" movement. Although I loved the ideas, I eventually accepted that I could keep them in mind but with a husband, a dog, a job, and 5 kids my life just wasn't destined to be simple. My current day-to-day routines make me feel like what I actually have is involuntary complexity. I try to be conscious of keeping my actions in line with my values and of accepting the richness of my complicated life. Right now, the involuntary complexity of my day-to-day routines is tiring but I have good people on my team trying to help me get to a cancer-free life that is worth living. It is SO unfair that I am here receiving the best care the world has to offer and people in Sierra Leone right now get nothing.

One of the many challenges to my sense of myself has been accepting ingesting poison, and intermittently being "toxic." This was a regular part of the hospital experience and I am now toxic at home. As someone who has tried to live a healthy life in some kind of harmony with nature, I had to remind myself early on that "chemo" does do some good things if you're lucky. It doesn't feel great to have people caring for you need to be in gowns, masks, gloves etc to protect themselves from you but it's all part of trying to get to a better place.

The most recent blow has been having vision problems. For someone like me, not being able to read is a BIG deal. Unfortunately, I am on high dose prednisone and that can cause blurry vision. I will be surprised if I am not also developing graft-versus-host-disease in my eyes. I hope to see an eye doctor soon to learn about treatment options. The tacrolimus I take to suppress my immune system makes my hands tremulous and I am jittery and scatter-brained since beginning prednisone. I am doing all I can in terms of diet and exercise to minimize my bone loss and muscle wasting. I am so focused on function that I find I am mostly able to accept the ongoing assaults to my physical appearance.

Quite a few friends and family have caught themselves complaining to me about things like job stress and then apologized, noting that they aren't going through anything like what we are. I'd like it recorded in the minutes that I have NO waning interest in your lives or global events—just very little time at the moment to attend to anything beyond my body. I WANT to hear how things really are for you. A number of people have mentioned that our experience has shifted their perspective on their own lives, rooted them a bit more in the present and increased their appreciation of small pleasures. It adds meaning to our suffering to know that our experience might in some ways enrich the lives of others.

Dave continues to soldier on in good spirits in spite of every day being chores from dawn to dusk. We both laugh now at having thought that during this recovery time we might be able to catch up on reading or watch a few movies. Neither of us has done either one. The basic tasks, ever changing meds and routines, and the emotional toll of the vast uncertainty ahead leave us both totally exhausted by early evening. Even so, I am grateful that in the midst of all this I feel completely like myself. I am still here, not unraveling, and intend to survive, hopefully thrive.

I wish the very best for all of you and can't thank you enough for the love and encouragement during this epic trek.

Love,
Kathryn

THE MATHEMATICS OF RECOVERY

Dave

October 4' 2014

Day +70: I grew up in a rather dour Scottish family where praise was discouraged. It was frowned upon, even. Because, as I am sure you know, if you praise someone it will simply go to their head and make them conceited and lazy. And celebrations? Don't get me started on celebrations. They should be few and far between and should be muted and quiet if they happen at all. We wouldn't want the neighbors to think we were full of ourselves, would we? And in any case, just when you start celebrating, life has a habit of making something bad happen to you soon thereafter just to bring you down a peg or two and remind you of the folly of celebrating or looking on the bright side. So in eleventh grade, for example, when everyone took the national standardized exams that would determine whether you could go on to university or other career paths several kids in our neighborhood got new bikes just for **passing** their exams. And I'm not talking about boring, heavy, Raleigh bikes with 3-speed Sturmey-Archer gears and saddle bags - I'm talking about fancy lightweight Peugeot racing bikes with 12-speed French gears, thin tires and drop down handles! So what did I get for getting an A in every single exam and being top of the class? I got a firm handshake and a stern look from my father. He then, much against his better judgment I am sure, muttered the following sentence. It is still ringing in my ears 45 years later...

"Aye, well, I don't suppose you could do much better than that."

Praise indeed! Now you can see where my sunny nature and cheery disposition comes from.

I mention all this this because I want to share some updates with you but I am aware that many of the people who are reading these journal entries are... how can I put this delicately?... are **Americans**. Americans just brimming with irrational enthusiasm and overflowing with ill-advised optimism! You might overreact to what I am about to share but I'll need to take the chance.

Some of Kathryn's lab results and numbers are IMPROVING! Several of them, in fact. Her liver function tests, which have been worrying us for quite some time, are definitely trending down in a good direction. I took some convincing, and had to graph it out to be quite sure. It is unclear what has caused the improvement. It could be the prednisone or the beclomethasone-in-corn-oil or some combination of those and other unknown things but there is no doubt that they are on their way back down towards normal. Our team at SCCA is convinced enough that they are starting a slow taper of Kathryn's prednisone over the next couple of months. Of course there could be many more ups and downs ahead of us. Kathryn is still on a ton of different medications and infusions. Her prednisone dose might have to go back up again at some point. She still has significant GVHD affecting her eyes and mouth, among other things, but this is a big step forward. And her hemoglobin (red cells), white cells and platelets are better than they have been in a decade! Our transplant team doctors and nurses can't tell us how long her recovery will take and how healthy and well she will feel at any stage along the way but they do say that she is doing better than 95% of people they deal with who are at this stage (Day +70) in the recovery process.

So how is Kathryn reacting to this news? The other day when we were trudging up and down the stairs in Discovery Park she remarked that it felt as though the journey we were on was a bit like climbing Mount Everest. And that got me thinking. Mount Everest is about 29,000 feet high (give or take a snowdrift or two). But the stairs we were climbing are, on average only 8 inches high. So in order to climb Mount Everest we would need to climb 29,000 X 12/8 or 43,500 steps. And since those steps are in flights of 12 + 5 + 5 + 4 + 5 + 5 + 5 + 5 + 4 + 5 + 5 + 5 + 5 + 5 + 6 + 5 + 25 for a total of 111 Kathryn suggested that if we went up and down 9 times and then stepped up on the first step and back down once more that would be (9 X 111) + 1 = 1000 steps which would be much easier to count and if we did that for 43.5 days then we would have climbed a "Mount-

Everest-worth" of steps. **Let's do that!** I know I am probably oversharing a bit, here, but those are the kind of sappy, romantic conversations that Kathryn and I have with each other these days.

It is likely to be another year or longer before we feel that Kathryn is getting close to a stable post-transplant state of health (with her IV central line gone and being off most of her medications) but it now feels mathematically more likely than not that we will get to that day. And when we do we could host a demure, muted gathering and invite all of you to come. We wouldn't even need to call it a celebration. We could hold it on a dull, cloudy day so that the neighbors could see that we weren't really having any fun. And each of you could walk up to Kathryn, give her a stern look and a firm handshake and say:

"Aye, well, I don't suppose you could do much better than that."

On second thought... to hell with that! We'll have a great, rowdy celebration on a warm sunny summer's day. And since I am now an American citizen I can be as obnoxiously loud and as irrationally optimistic as I like! I can praise Kathryn for her unrelenting patience and perseverance throughout all of this and we can both be thankful for the love and support we have received from so many people along the way. And I don't care what our neighbors might think. Actually most of our neighbors are really nice. We'll invite them too.

Now **that's** something to look forward to!

DAY 80 EVALUATION

Kathryn

October 12, 2014

Next week I have 14 appointments. At around Day 80 transplant patients have a variety of exams to assess their current status and advise them about care needs and what to watch out for over the coming months. Dave and I are making transitions in our daily routines that will allow me to manage more on my own as he returns to work. I know I will still have his tremendous love and support but it will be an adjustment for him to dive back into work and for me to spend a lot of time at home alone.

Prior to the onset of graft-versus-host-disease and beginning prednisone, I felt well enough to be asking all of you for ideas about things to do around Seattle that I may have never had time for. I felt quite good and imagined I would have some time to do some of them. As it has turned out, the requirements of each day (right now four IV infusions at home) are so time consuming that we haven't done a single thing on the terrific list of ideas that you all shared. I will keep it though with hopes of doing some of them over the coming year. I began this treatment with the idea that I would have to pay with a year of my life, in hopes of living quite a few more. It requires me to focus on myself and my body in a way that does not feel natural to me but I want to maximize the chances of doing well over time.

I will be forever grateful to my donor and my "Jersey girls" for creating healthy blood cells for me and I want to think of them as my friends. I now have good counts of red cells, white cells, and platelets, and that's what I signed up for. It seems like a paradox that these same cells are the ones assaulting previously healthy parts of my body in harmful ways that require treatment with very unpleasant side effects.

Although overall things seem to be moving in the right direction, I felt much better 6-8 weeks ago than I feel now. I have 31 pills to take today and I now have trembling hands, feel like I can't think straight, am jittery, and have blurry vision. Because of the prednisone, my face and belly are getting rounder and my arms and legs are disappearing in spite of getting regular exercise. This, plus the demands of each day, does not allow me to be in touch personally with my friends and family in the ways that I would like to be.

I am aware that I have made a mental shift that feels good in my thinking about my future. A friend recently texted me from a store asking if I wanted her to pick up a pair of pants for me. After the text exchange, I realized that even though I don't need pants right now, I am assuming I will live to need another pair of pants. Last spring, I was about to buy some pants and then had the thought that it might be a waste of money if I didn't live through the fall, so I returned them to the shelf. I had thoroughly read about the many possible risks and complications of transplants and knew there were no guarantees. Although there still aren't, I **AM** planning on being alive in a year.

Although this is the hardest thing I've ever done by a factor of 100, I give thanks each day for all of your support, my loving husband, my wonderful kids, my home and garden, and not having to contemplate financial ruin as I try to recover. I so wish that all people going through this process could have my good fortune.

Best wishes to all of you as the leaves fall and the holiday season draws near.

Love,
Kathryn

EARLY MORNING WAKE UP CALL

Dave

October 17, 2014

Day +83: Kathryn and I have heard from seasoned "transplanters" several times during the past few months that "...everyone has set backs and ups and downs during the first 100 days. Most people need to be readmitted at least once for a fever or some such thing." So I guess we were pushing our cosmic luck to think that we might sneak through without such an event. Apparently not...

At about 1am this morning Kathryn felt some tightness in her chest and had a fast and irregular pulse. She felt a little dizzy and slightly breathless. No real chest pain, no jaw or arm pain or other more worrying signs like sweating. It didn't get better after half an hour of sitting up and drinking cold water and warm tea so we talked to the on-call SCCA triage nurse, and as I suspected, she recommended that I bring Kathryn to the UW Emergency Department. They confirmed that Kathryn's heart was in Atrial flutter/ fibrillation with a heart rate of about 160 beats per minute and slightly low blood pressure. They gave her 20mg of a drug called diltiazem which brought her back into normal rhythm with a rate of around 70 in just a couple of minutes and she has stayed in that rhythm ever since. Her ECG looked otherwise quite normal. Both her magnesium and potassium levels are low (which is a side effect of some of her meds) and that is the likely cause for the arrhythmia. They are giving her IV potassium and magnesium and have started her on a low dose of metoprolol (a pill that will keep her heart rate from going up so high). They will probably keep her in for a day or maybe two and check to make sure she didn't damage her heart (but I think that is highly unlikely) and be sure that nothing else is going on.

She is up on 8NE (the transplant unit floor above the one where she spent her 24 days in July/August) at UWMC, since 8NE has better intensive care facilities should Kathryn need those. She has her phone and laptop with her but she is trying to nap right now. She is fully alert and feels fine and is annoyed that she is causing everyone so much bother! The attending physician on the unit is the charming and bright Brazilian doctor whom we had met while Kathryn was in getting her transplant in July. The "mid-level" was another of our favorite staff members, a nurse practitioner called Joanne who was very thorough, thoughtful, and knowledgeable. Both of them came beaming into

Kathryn's room and said how great she looked and how pleased they were to see her again (albeit under less than ideal circumstances, they added!). "We almost never get to see people again who are doing as well as you!"

For the medically inclined readers of our journal the consensus is that this is a common arrhythmia post transplant and that it may have been precipitated by Kathryn's low magnesium and potassium level. All of this is correctable. Her cardiac enzyme (troponin) levels were normal which indicates that there has been no damage to her heart muscle. They will keep her in overnight tonight but if things continue like this she will likely be discharged back home tomorrow or Sunday.

Let's hope that this is just a bump in the road. We actually got some good news during the week. Kathryn's heart exam and lung function tests were excellent and her DEXA scan (measuring bone density) didn't look as bad as expected, so our worries about osteoporosis, while still there, are somewhat less concerning to us right now. The plan is to continue to slowly taper Kathryn off her prednisone but to continue most of the other drugs and the infusions of electrolytes for several more weeks or months.

ENOUGH WITH THE DRAMA

Kathryn

October 20, 2014

We were hoping to be on Vashon this past weekend but instead got to spend it at UW Hospital and SCCA. Luckily, I almost always find difficulty ***interesting*** at least, and a middle of the night trip to an ER was a new experience. I really didn't feel all that bad given that my usual heart rate is in the low 60's and it was 161 by the time we got to the ER. It seemed prudent to go in and it's good that we did. They kept me overnight and I was discharged Saturday.

We weren't thrilled about having to go to SCCA appointments the day after discharge on a sunny Sunday but got some good news. We have been watching my liver function tests as I taper my prednisone with hopes that they don't rise again and I don't have worsening of my graft-versus-host-disease symptoms. My labs are still going in the right direction. We were also told that my bone marrow biopsy from last week showed no trace of disease. My chimerism is 100%, meaning it's all my "Jersey girl" cells, and not my previous unhealthy cells, that are in there, and they are doing what they are supposed to do in the blood department. I just have to accept some amount of GVHD as the price I pay. My bone density has not been good in the past so I've been worried about losing more bone due to being on high dose prednisone. We also got my DEXA report a few days ago and to my astonishment my bone density seems to be less bad than they expected. I am not yet convinced that the report I received is actually mine (!)

Our weekend was brightened by a surprise visit home from Murray. Since our 5 kids, spouses and grandkids (15 people at the moment) are spread all over the country, we rarely manage to have everyone at home at once. It was great to have both Cameron and Murray here on such an eventful weekend. Hadley, one of our dear granddaughters, also sent me a card saying she couldn't wait to see me out of the hospital "all nice and new :-)"

I have various tests and appointments over the next two weeks and will then be discharged back to Group Health, with support from the Long Term Follow-Up group at SCCA. I am grateful that my doctor and I will have their expertise as a resource for the rest of my life. I hope I don't need them much.

Dave and I feel ready for him to return to work and for me to manage more of my recovery at home. I have been told that I will need to be patient and focus my efforts on recovering in the months to come. We are hopeful that I will gradually feel better and better over that time.

Hope you are all finding time to savor these glorious autumn days, rain or shine.

Love,
Kathryn

"OCH, YE'LL NO' MELT!"

Dave

October 22, 2014

Day +88: One of the attributes on the **very** long list of things that I adore about Kathryn Crawford is her indomitable spirit. Some people might call it incomprehensible stubbornness or just plain lunacy but I prefer to categorize it as her indomitable spirit. There is never a question about whether or not we are going to go for our daily four-mile-walk-plus-stair-trudging. The only questions are about when it might be best to fit it in on a particular day and whether we might need to make any adjustments to how we go about it. So this morning we awoke to a good solid northwest autumn downpour. One and a half inches fell overnight along with wind gusting to 40 miles per hour. The rain showed no signs of letting up all day - a glorious, steady, robust, bouncing-off-the-sidewalk, earth-replenishing deluge. As we peered through the grey sheets of water lashing off our neighbors' roofs we could barely make out the trees of Discovery Park in the distance.

Time for a reality check.

"Hey, Dave, let's get up early and get my gancyclovir infusion going right now to give us more time to get ready for our walk."

That was no problem. Gancyclovir is one of the little "hand grenades" that self-deflates in about an hour so we did that while we had breakfast and did morning chores. But how to deal with the saline, magnesium, and phosphate infusion... that one needs to be connected to the portable battery-operated infusion pump ("Darth Vader in a handbag"). We wouldn't want water to get in and short-circuit the pump!

"No problem, I'll just put the pump inside its own little backpack, put all of that a inside a plastic bag, and then I can put ALL of that inside my regular back pack when we go for our walk!"

That was easy, too. There is no shortage of plastic bags in the Crawford-McCulloch household these days since I seem to go to Bartells every other day for plastic gloves, alcohol swabs, creams, potions, eye drops, mouth washes...

"But what about my head? How do I deal with my bald head? Will it feel too cold or too hot, I wonder? How will I keep it dry?"

No-o-o-o problem to our ever-resourceful Kathryn. She took a fleece-beanie skullcap, a headscarf, a plastic shower cap, and then covered that with a hooded oilskin jacket, waterproof pants and rubber boots. Yes, the prep work for our walk was a little more involved today than it often is but, hey, look on the bright side, we really didn't need to slather SPF-50 sunscreen over every square inch of Kathryn's body today since barely half a square inch was actually exposed to the elements. So there we were an hour later trudging around the Loop Trail, laughing, chatting, and listening to the wind howling, watching the leaves blowing across the path and doing our best impression of Tim Robbins in the Shawshank Redemption when we got to any really big puddles! We probably looked like alien lunatics who had escaped from captivity but you'll be astonished to hear that we didn't pass a single other person during the walk so no-one got to see us! We were careful not to slip on wet leaves as we went up and down the stairs and got back to the house soaked to the skin and grinning from ear to ear a couple of hours later.

My grandfather would have approved. Wullie McCulloch was not a man to let a little rain interfere with his life. Wullie worked as a metal lathe machinist in Jack's Metal Factory in Maybole, Ayrshire, and lived in a small council house nearby with my granny. Every summer we would drive to Maybole to spend a couple of weeks with them. And since Scottish summer holidays include many rainy days there were occasions when, by the middle of the morning, three rambunctious little boys were getting under grampa's feet and interfering with his reading of the morning paper.

"Away ye go outside and get rid of yer energy out there!"

"But grampa, it's po-o-o-o-o-ouring with rain!"

Wullie would glance above the top of the newspaper and scowl at the rivers of water streaming down the outside of the window.

"A wee skiddle of rain will no' hurt ye!" he would

pronounce, and then say, for added emphasis, **"Och, ye'll no' melt!"**

And out I would go. He was right, of course. Even though my vivid five-year-old imagination thought that I would dissolve into a slimy puddle of skin, bones and guts that would slowly seep into the grass so that I would disappear never to be seen again... that never actually happened. I would bounce back into the house a couple of hours later with rosy cheeks and a huge appetite for whatever stick-to-your-ribs soup granny had made for lunch.

As I look back I am glad that I did not melt and disappear back in Scotland when I was five. Because of that, and because of thousands upon thousands of other unlikely events I have ended up fifty-some years later walking and laughing through Discovery Park in Seattle with this incredible woman. The chances that she and I would ever cross paths seems so unlikely, looking back, that I still find myself pinching myself for the good fortune of getting to have Kathryn in my life.

Thanks for giving me good advice and a good attitude, grampa. It has served me well.

CONFESSIONS OF A WEARY TRAVELER

Dave

October 27, 2014

Day +93: I hesitated about writing anything today. I am not feeling particularly optimistic or upbeat and I don't really have anything new to report, so why write at all? I am sure many of you are sick of getting these seemingly never-ending updates of tedious medical appointments and lab values and new symptoms. However much you love Kathryn and me you are getting on with your own busy lives and maybe looking forward to the celebration that we hope will happen at sometime in the future. I can assure you that Kathryn and I are also sick of the never-ending updates. But in order to help me understand what I am feeling and why, I want to document and understand the mood I'm in today.

Yesterday marked exactly three months since the stem cells from "Jersey" were infused in to Kathryn's body. So how did we celebrate that event? Not with cake, nor with a glass of non-alcoholic sparkling beverage, I'm afraid. Instead we shared a weary sigh and did an inventory of all the things that we need to accomplish this week in order to make it possible for Kathryn's recovery to continue when I get back to work next Monday on **Day +100**. It has been a 16 hours a day effort for both of us for every single one of these last 93 days just keeping up with everything we need to attend to and deal with to keep Kathryn on a healing path. While I love my work and am eager to get back to the work itself, and to the many friends and colleagues whom I interact with there, I have some apprehension about how it will feel for me and even more about how it will feel for Kathryn.

We have used the analogy of a journey throughout this narrative for obvious reasons. We are on a re-e-e-e-eally long journey and are entering a tedious, boring part. In my mind I sometimes think of it as being like a long cross-country road trip. Many of you, I am sure, have embarked on long road trips at some point in your lives. I often enjoy them immensely, which has got me to wondering why I am not enjoying this particular "road trip" the way I often do. I have imagined this journey as traveling east-to-west across this great country of ours. Since I much prefer the Northwest to anywhere else I have traveled within the USA I have imagined that our journey started off in some noisy, bustling city on the East coast where there was constant noise, aggressive driving, toll roads, flashing lights, and a constant sense of danger. That is kind of how it felt when Kathryn was in the UW transplant unit! But now we have struggled through the maze of turnpikes, roundabouts, speed traps and traffic jams and have gotten ourselves onto I-90 heading west. The ultimate destination, for me, is in a warm comfy house on lovely, quiet Vashon Island in the beautiful Pacific Northwest where the proportion of Nature-to-People-to-Concrete is more to my liking. I am headed there with the love of my life hoping to enjoy many, many years of adventures there with her using that as our base. With that analogy in mind I guess that right now we are maybe somewhere in Indiana heading west.

So why am I not having more fun?

On a regular road trip there are many things that you can enjoy. If you basically feel well and have no aches and pains or discomforts, and you are not bursting to go to the bathroom, there is something soothing about traveling on endless miles of US highway. You know where you are going. You know roughly when you will get there. If you change your mind you can turn around and go back, or you can take an off ramp and pick a new destination. If you are in a reliable car you don't need to worry about anything breaking down. If it is a modern, comfortable car you can keep your temperature not-too-hot and not-too-cold. You can stock up on junk food and pop, and justify it to yourself that there weren't better options available at the 7-11 in Podunk, Nebraska, and that you can get back on your diet and eat healthier when you get to your destination. Your car probably has a built-in entertainment system so that, if you feel so inclined, you could listen to every single album that Dick Gaughan or Tom Waits ever wrote... in chronological order... belting out the melodies along with the stereo with no-one holding their ears or yelling at you to shut up! Or for a change of pace you could listen to a nice thriller or adventure story narrated by a suave, intelligent, reassuring English actor as the corn fields and soy fields drift by on either side. There are signposts letting you know when the next gas station or restaurant or motel is coming up so you can just pace yourself and make easy decisions depending on how the mood takes you...

WALL DRUG AHEAD IN 642 MILES!

And then, as a great example of American highway humor you'll see another huge signpost about 100 miles later saying...

WHAT THE HECK IS WALL DRUG?

With the right attitude and good company long cross-country road trips are awesome...

But that is not what this "road trip" feels like for Kathryn or me, right now. It feels like we have woken up in the middle of a really bad episode of the Twilight Zone. Kathryn's basic level of day-to-day comfort is not very high. She has lots of aches and pains and irritations in her eyes and mouth and skin so that it is hard to truly relax. She feels weak, jittery and with a foggy brain. If our "destination" is some new stable steady state of health then it is unclear exactly where that destination is or how long it will take to get there or indeed what it will feel like when we do get there. And it seems like we drifted off to sleep and woke up on a different road. This doesn't feel like I-90 anymore. There are no off ramps so we can't turn around and go back and we can't choose a different destination. We just need to keep going along this unfriendly and unfamiliar road and hope that it begins to feel more familiar at some point. We could be in Indiana... or maybe Minnesota, or South Dakota... they all look about the same. The skies seem black and foggy up ahead on the horizon and we have a sense of foreboding that maybe a Funnel Cloud could be forming and coming our way in the future. And the car we are traveling in doesn't seem all that reliable either. It is like a 1986 Corolla with 340,000 miles on it. There are squeaks and rattles that didn't used to be there. We have been told to inspect the outside of the car regularly to see if new holes or patches of rust appear but it is unclear what we are supposed to do about it if we find them. The ride is bumpy and uncomfortable, the front left struts seem to be failing and the radio is broken so there is not much to entertain us along the way. The gas gauge is broken, too, so it is unclear how much gas is in our tank. And there aren't any reassuring signposts on this strange road so we don't know what lies ahead for us. Nothing says:

HAPPY VALLEY AHEAD IN 214 DAYS!

or

PEOPLE WHO GET THIS FAR USUALLY END UP DOING FINE!

I hope that Kathryn will write more at some point about how it feels to have this constant lack of reassurance that accompanies us on this journey. The staff at the UW transplant unit and at SCCA are friendly and competent and tell us that Kathryn is "doing great" but never acknowledge that what they consider "doing great" is not what this wonderful, vibrant, complex, layered individual would have considered "doing great" a year or so ago. It makes us wonder just where the bar is set. She is bald, tremulous with lots of bodily irritations, and difficulty concentrating or sleeping while she juggles 30+ pills every day plus intravenous infusions and clinic schedules. We get no reassurance that if we keep doing everything as fastidiously and reliably as we have been for the past 93 days that things will eventually get significantly easier or better. We just get constantly changing lists of things we need to do and drugs we need to take to keep moving forward.

So forgive me if I am not feeling too chipper today. Kathryn and I will continue to limp along this long, lonely unfamiliar highway and hope that we will get to a good destination and more familiar and reassuring sights eventually. We both appreciate immensely the love and support that you are all giving us. We know that, if you could, you would get out and shove the car for us if it would get us to a happy destination sooner.

Is that a break in the clouds up ahead with some sun shining through? Maybe we are closer to Montana than we thought. After that we go through Idaho and then drop down into Washington. You know Corollas are VERY reliable. If we just keep going we should get there. I happen to know that there are a lot of friendly people waiting there to welcome us.

Let's just take another deep breath, Kath, and keep going...

MAYBE I SHOULD EXPRESS GLOOMY PESSIMISM AND FRUSTRATION MORE OFTEN!

Dave

October 31, 2014

Day +97: Two days after my last gloomy ***Confessions of a weary traveler*** journal entry we had our "Transition Conference" at SCCA. This is where the attending physician and nurse on our SCCA team (the "Tan" team) reviewed all the results of the 80-day evaluation and reflected on how Kathryn has done and then gave us clear instructions about what should happen over the next 3-9 months as Kathryn transitions to get most of her care back at Group Health (before she comes back for another week of 1-year evaluations at SCCA next July). They gave us a copy of the letter that will be sent to Kathryn's oncologist and also to her primary care provider summarizing the hardest four months of our lives into a few succinct paragraphs of medico-jargon! For the medically inclined who may be interested in exactly what they said I will reprint it here. I will then give a translation that should make more sense to everyone else:

Ms. Crawford's date of transplant was July 26, 2014. She received cyclophsohamide 120mg/kg and busulfan that was targeted to 800 to 900 ng/mL followed by infusion of the PBSC. Her GVHD prophylaxis consisted of tacrolimus and methotrexate.

We reviewed the transplant course and discussed the following topics:

1. Graft status and chimerism: Her most recent CBC on October 27th, 2014 show a white blood count of 4.9, hemoglobin 13.6, hematocrit 39, and her platelet count was 145,000. On differential, her absolute neutrophil count was 3.62. Her chimerism in her blood showed CD3 was 100% donor and CD33 was 100% donor on October 14, 2014. The patients ABO blood type was A- and the donor A+. Her last blood transfusion was 8/6/2014 and platelet transfusion was 8/4/2014. Should she require transfusions, the products should be irradiated and leukoreduced.

2. Disease status: Her bone marrow performed on October 14, 2014, showed hypocellularity without evidence of disease, though there were still large areas of loose stromal fibrosis along with the focal trilineage hypoplasia. Her cytogenetics were normal, though she had no preceding cytogenetic marker. Flow cytometry had no evidence of disease. On her JAK2 test done on her peripheral blood on October 23, 2014, no mutation was detected, whereas pretransplant her study was

positive for the JAK2 mutation.

3. GVHD and recommendations for ongoing immune suppression.

(A) Acute: Following transplant, the patient had a variety of presumed GVHD issues which began approximately 35 to 40 days post transplant. She developed a rash on her upper chest and shoulders with severe pruritus. A skin biopsy on September 2, 2014, did not conclusively diagnose GVHD as there is a keratonotic dysplasia caused by busulfan toxicity or GVHD. She was treated topically and with PUVA, though she developed significant oral changes that were consistent with oral GVHD. She also had transaminitis which was attributed to medications, though they continued to progress despite stopping the medications thought to be responsible. GI was consulted, and this was thought to be a liver GVHD. Therefore, in the setting of skin, oral, and presumed liver GVHD, she was treated initially with 0.5 mg/kg of prednisone starting on September 9, 2014. Because her LFTs continued to increase, the prednisone was increased to 1mg/kg. Because her liver function tests did not significantly decrease GI service recommended starting high-dose beclomethasone, which was initiated on September 20, 2014, which coincided with improvement of her liver function tests. She eventually was able to be initiated on a steroid taper, which has been tolerated and is scheduled to be completed on November 20, 2014.

Translation:

Her blood counts (the red cells, white cells and platelets) are coming 100% from the new donor stem cells and are in the "stellar" normal range. There is no evidence of her previous disease whatsoever (they expect to still see some fibrosis in the bone marrow at this stage but that will likely continue to get cleaned out by the new stem cells over the next several months). Her liver function tests are almost normal, her kidney function is normal, and they see nothing that alarms them.

So that is the miraculous part of all of this. They then proceeded to throw a LARGE bucket of cold water and caveats on all of this using language that sounds alarming even if you don't understand what all the words mean. They gave the following advice for the Group Health doctors who will be following Kathryn's progress from here in one single sentence of terrifying medico-jargon:

Please monitor for progression of GVHD which may be manifested by sclerotic skin changes and lichen planus skin eruptions, erythematous maculopapular rashes, hair loss, premature gray hair, onychodystrophy/ lysis, ocular sicca/oral sicca/oral sensitivity/oral lichenoid changes/oral ulcers and dysphagia with esophageal strictures, dyspnea with obstructive and restrictive lung defects, liver function test abnormalities, nausea, vomiting, diarrhea, weight loss, fasciitis, joint contractures, serositis, dyspareunia, among others...

Translation:

A-a-a-a-a-all righty, then! Just about any part of Kathryn's body could still come under attack at any time so stay alert to all possibilities and don't let your guard down or relax for a moment!

Actually when we asked pointed questions of the "Tan" team doctor and nurse they made it clear that they think Kathryn not only **HAS** done incredibly well up to this point but that they think she is **GOING** to do well moving forward. Yes, her magnesium level is still on the low side so they want her to continue to get magnesium infusions through the Hickman central IV line for a few more weeks but after that the central line can be removed and she can get her magnesium supplements in pill form. Her cytomegalovirus (CMV) viral counts are back to undetectable levels and so the (antiviral) gancyclovir hand grenades can be stopped right now. They acknowledged that Kathryn has had GVHD affecting her skin, liver, eyes, and mouth but that these are all under good control and have been minor and grumbling rather than explosive and severe in how they have come on or progressed. For those reasons they recommended that her prednisone should be tapered off and stopped completely in the next four weeks so that she will continue with tacrolimus as her sole immunosuppressive for the next 9 months. She will continue on an antibiotic and antiviral (both in pill form) for the next 9 months at least, but the antifungal can be stopped once she is off prednisone. They all think that her heart fluttering episode was a minor thing related to the low magnesium levels and that she should continue on the metoprolol (to keep the heart rate from getting too fast) for another couple of months at which time a Group Health cardiologist can evaluate her and decide if that, too, can be stopped. The acid-suppressing drug (pantoprazole) which has helped with acid reflux and abdominal discomfort related to taking all these pills can also be stopped once Kathryn is off the prednisone.

In other words we **DO** see signs that the number of meds (infusions through central IV lines and pills) are all likely to be decreasing over the next few weeks, which will lead to a greater sense of normalcy for Kathryn and me. Yes, it is possible that Kathryn might experience a relapse in any of her GVHD symptoms or might get new signs and symptoms related to GVHD or it is possible that she could develop new infections but none of those things is all that likely so they feel comfortable reducing her meds.

So we will proceed with cautious optimism, although part of me thinks that I should express my gloomy pessimism and frustration more often since we got all of this "good news" two days after my last gloomy Caring Bridge rant! Maybe I should throw in some grumpiness and bad temper just for good measure!

WHAT'S THE DRILL?

Kathryn

November 12, 2014

This expression always makes me think of Dave's dad. He used to ask that question when he wondered what the plan was for the day when he was vacationing here from Scotland. When could he expect lunch to be served? Would there be an outing or an event to look forward to? What should he expect during the day?

When I set up our Caring Bridge site I really didn't have much idea how we would use it - what we'd write here, how often, etc. I assumed that it would probably be brief updates and that Dave and I would both be writing our own personal notes about our experience elsewhere. As it has turned out, neither of us has really had time to write anything elsewhere so Caring Bridge will be our record of what this experience has been like. It will be great to also have a record of the love and support from all of you.

This past week Dave returned to work and I continued trying to figure out how my complicated regimen was going to work at Group Health. I had made the required number of doctor appointments but I also need regularly delivered, and ever changing, IVs, all the related tubing and tapes, and central line dressing change supplies. We have been using a delivery company that does "just in time" deliveries and is very reliable. It has been a rocky week but I should have it figured out in another week or so. Dave is glad to be back at work and it feels good to him to reconnect with colleagues.

I am continuing the taper off my prednisone and will be elated if I actually get off of it on my first taper. Frequently, as people taper the dose, the graft-versus-host-disease symptoms worsen and the dose has to go back up. I am really hoping this doesn't happen since my biggest quality of life issues at the moment are drug-related blurry vision, irritated eyes, feeling sort of scatter brained, and muscle weakness. The eye irritation is related to GVHD in my eyes but the blur seems to be improving as my prednisone dose goes down. I feel like I can cope with a lot if I can see and think.

I now have my first cold since my new immune system was installed. I don't feel well but I seem to be slowly getting better. I have learned a lot about vulnerability and accepting help during this experience. I have relied on Dave more than I would ever have imagined and he has almost convinced me that he doesn't mind being in the role of my caregiver. The whole experience has been just about as demanding for him as for me, just in different ways. Over the coming year I must continue to be aware of the ways in which I am vulnerable, particularly now that cold and flu season is here. I knew from the beginning that I would much rather be the nurse than the patient (!)

Although I miss feeling like I am part of the world in a productive and giving way, I am trying to accept that right now this is how it must be for me in order to maximize my chances of a good recovery. Exercise is more important than ever as I try to regain the strength and muscle lost during this time on prednisone. Although Dave suggested in a recent post that I have an indomitable spirit, I really don't. I feel pretty tough most of the time but have days where I just feel like I'm being pushed down into the mud and need a good cry.

This week I experimented with wearing a mask at the grocery store, not because it protects *me* but because I've been told that others would keep their distance. I was actually struck by two things. Lots of people seemed not to even really notice, and others were particularly helpful, offering to run and get something I forgot while I was at the cashier. There are a lot of wonderful people out there.

I am also figuring out how I want to keep my bald head warm. I've just been relying on simple bandanas but they aren't very warm and don't stay put with a coat and hood. I bought a cut-rate wig early on since I thought I might want one when the weather cooled. It doesn't look too bad and stays put more easily than scarves. One of the umpteen problems I am supposed to monitor over the next couple of years is hair loss. I look forward to the day when that might apply to me. In the meantime I will be monitoring for hair reappearance :-)

Soon Murray will be home from school for

Thanksgiving and we're really looking forward to having him here with Cameron, and also Wendy and family. Everyone has gotten flu shots and we will give them a serious refresher on hand washing and covering coughs. The holidays will be unusual this year with hardly any family around, and maybe not even a tree and the greens that I love so much. We can still have all the homemade cookies that I usually bake, though, and I will be happy to be at home.

More than one post-transplant patient I talked to mentioned that recovery is really a marathon and not a sprint. Dave and I are really feeling that and, in some ways, the intense experience of the hospital was easier because we knew it would end. Now that we are into the long slog part, I expect that we will be writing here somewhat less. I am sorry that I haven't been able to be in touch with more people individually but it just hasn't been possible.

So "What's the drill for me, these days?" Hand-washing, eye drops, pill-counting, careful food preparation, clinic-scheduling, supply-ordering, walking, weight training, IV infusion hook-ups, pill-swallowing, IV infusion disconnects, tedious-shower-preparation, rinse-and-repeat... Unfortunately, I don't really look forward to meals all that much. Since my taste buds aren't quite right and I have sores in my mouth I've come to see food more as vehicles for getting pills down and keeping my protein intake up to fend off some of the prednisone-induced muscle wasting. Most of my "outings" and "events" revolve around lab visits and clinic appointments with breaks for meals. Even so, I do feel like I am making slow progress and am on my way to a better place. I am savoring every one of these glorious sunny days and crossing my fingers for some snow this winter. My life is not anything like it was a year ago but I am most grateful that I am still here.

We cherish all the love and support we continue to receive from all of you. It has made all the difference in keeping our spirits up. Many thanks.

Love,

Kathryn

ALL QUIET ON THE PREDNISONE FRONT

Dave

December 1, 2014

Day +128: As the Thanksgiving weekend comes to an end I could easily fill several pages with all the sappy, sentimental things that I am thankful for, because it really is a long list... but that would make for tedious, predictable, and unoriginal reading, so I won't do that. On this the most unusual and challenging year of Kathryn's life and of mine let me, instead, share a few of the less commonplace and predictable things for which I am thankful...

I am thankful that although Kathryn has lost her hair she has not lost her sense of humor. I will say that her sense of humor (and mine) has been sorely tested these past ten months but for the most part humor (gallows and otherwise) has helped us to keep things in perspective and to find comfort and some amusement in the absurd. And I can share with you some *Breaking News* that a dark brown "peach fuzz" has reappeared on the adorable shiny bald Kathronian head in the past week and is gradually getting easier to see so that is something else to be thankful for. How fast it grows and what it ends up looking like is just something else that we both need to keep a good sense of humor about but I see this as a positive sign.

I am thankful that Kathryn has had a Hickman central line in her chest for the past four and a half months... and that it has remained patent and uninfected for all of that time... but that she won't need to have it coming out of her chest forever. Okay that's a pretty long-winded and multi-layered expression of thanks. It is hard to imagine how Kathryn could have gotten through this without having excellent access to her big central veins for all of this time. Through those two lines she has received, by my estimation:

- 112 blood draws
- 470 infusions (everything from chemo drugs to antibiotics to blood and platelets and saline and electrolytes and nutrition...)
- 740 heparin flushes
- 1,345 saline flushes

This has also required 21 dressing changes, so far, and the end of each line (where the spring-loaded Clave sits) has been swabbed with alcohol around 2,700 times. Each of these events requires a nurse (or caregiver) to put on a fresh pair of gloves each time and to discard the packaging, plastic syringes, tubing, gauze swabs and empty bags of fluid afterwards so another thing that I am thankful for is that somewhere out in Eastern Washington there is a landfill with Kathryn's name on it.

I am thankful that Kathryn and I still seem to really enjoy each other's company despite being forced to spend 18+ hours every day involved in very intense, nerve-wracking, intimate-but-not-in-the-most-pleasant-sense activity with each other for over 130 days and counting... A lot of couples who are getting close to retirement begin to dread the arrival of that time in their lives because they will go from lives where they spent work days apart to a new time when they are forced to be together for wa-a-a-a-ay more hours every day than they have been used to. I feel that Kathryn and I have been able to do a dress rehearsal for our impending retirement (still probably about five years away for me) and that we "passed" that test. I never run out of things to talk about for which I'd love to hear Kathryn's take.

I am thankful that my days of washing individual spinach leaves (and even worse those finicky little leaves of curly kale with grooves and stems with bits of potentially-bacteria-encrusted-grit hiding in every nook and cranny) will be coming to an end in a few more months. In a spirit of trying to find something positive to say about this aspect of the past few months the fact that I have had to spend so much time carefully inspecting and washing and drying everything that is about to go into Kathryn's mouth has given me time to reflect on and have a new appreciation for where our food comes from and what it goes through between the field and the dinner plate. It has also given us a list of foods that Kathryn has not been able to have and so which we now crave (any soft cheeses like Brie, French pastries, tempeh, miso soup, or any unpacked foods from the deli, or anything that could have been touched and handled by other people's dirty hands).

I am thankful that my friends and colleagues at work still want to involve me in trying to transform healthcare for the better. These are fascinating times in American health care with rising costs and deteriorating outcomes becoming a growing crisis that we can't ignore. I have been back at work for four weeks now and am energized by what a positive impact we can all make by the work we do together. I am incredibly impressed with how much more Kathryn has been able to take on to make this possible for me. She has taken over most of the daily household chores, but since she still requires one or two infusions every day we now set our alarm for 4:30 or 5am every morning so that I can gently wake her, get an infusion set up, and then taken down an hour or two later before I have to take off for work.

I am REALLY thankful that Kathryn is no longer on Prednisone... at least for the moment. The delicate balance that we are trying to achieve over these next many months is to allow the new immune system to settle in and "do its thing" so that Kathryn gets the benefit of this (healthy numbers of red cells, white cells, platelets, and the ability to fight off infections and other outside "insults") while at the same time restraining the enthusiastic vigor of those new immune cells enough that they don't attack Kathryn's body in their spare time. For that she will remain on Tacrolimus for at least a year. Tacrolimus has side effects enough of its own (most notably causing tremulousness and magnesium deficiency). But Prednisone is added if graft-versus-host-disease becomes problematic. Kathryn was put on high doses of Prednisone for about six weeks and has slowly been tapered off it after that as GVH settled down. It was stopped altogether about ten days ago and so far things seem quiet and uneventful. We are hunkering down in our trenches staying vigilant for the signs that the enemy might be stirring out there ahead of us in the fog. We were both stunned at how quickly the side effects of high dose Prednisone became apparent (especially the round face and disappearing muscles) but are pleased to see those all reversing back towards normal.

I am thankful that the new immune system from the "Jersey girls" is doing a lot of things really well and is, for the most part, leaving Kathryn's body alone. Let's hope that continues long into 2015 and beyond...

I am thankful that we have a lot of exciting and happy things to look forward to in 2015. High on that list, for me, is that, after much deliberation, our plans to build a new house on our Vashon land are moving forward. It has also been a pleasant surprise, and something else for which I am thankful, just how much we enjoy our architect, Deborah, and our builder, Corey, and their families. It is truly fun to work with them on this project. All of our kids are also excited in anticipation of seeing the transformation coming about on this beautiful piece of quiet countryside.

I am thankful that the events of this past year have truly made me appreciate every single small delight in every day. Okay, that one was bordering on the sappy, sentimental and maudlin, so I'll move on quickly.

I am especially thankful that Kathryn Crawford continues to be the vital, vibrant, interesting,

unpredictable, loving, and delightful center of my life and will be for many years to come. Okay, McCulloch, that's enough. That one crosses the line. You need to finish this journal entry right now before people feel the need to reach for their Kleenex tissues or barf bags...

I hope that all of you enjoyed Thanksgiving and that you are looking forward to the rest of the Holiday season and the year ahead.

A DIFFERENT KIND OF JOURNEY

Kathryn

December 22, 2014

As we receive end of year letters from friends who have been on trips to far-flung places, I am struck by what a different kind of "trip" I have been on this year. Last spring, when I found out that I had a life threatening illness, I was asked several times if I was going to plan a big trip. My diagnosis did make me feel like a big trip was in order but it involved traveling into my own heart and spirit and mind, not around the world.

Although I have always tried to keep my actions lined up with my values, my experience this year has pushed me farther into contemplating my own mortality, what most adds meaning to my life, and what quality of life I might consider acceptable. It has forced me to live with vast uncertainty about what may unfold each day and to try my best to be grateful simply for the day that each sunrise brings. As Dave has walked with me every step of this trip, he has had a parallel experience of his own. For us as a couple, it has been a time of more connection and intimacy than ever before.

Dave may have jumped the gun a bit on celebrating the end of my prednisone prescription. It was delightful getting off of it and feeling like I could start trying to get my body back but 2-3 weeks after I stopped talking it, old and new signs of graft versus host disease appeared. I am now back on prednisone and will probably be on it for many months. This time I started at 30mg/day and, hopefully, I won't have to go higher. My eyes remain a problem that prednisone might make worse but they have seemed to be slowly improving.

After losing quite a bit of weight, I have worked my way back to 100lbs. I don't feel sturdy at this weight but am trying to be as active as I can. I feel like some kind of military recruit when I am on a treadmill with wrist weights and my central lines hanging off my front and my backpack with my IV hanging off my back. Exercise is really the only thing I can do to minimize the damage prednisone is doing to my muscles and bones.

Even though I would never wish what I have been through on anyone, Dave and I are aware of the many "gifts" we have received throughout the year. We have taken pleasure in being in touch with many people we don't normally have much contact with. We have learned a lot about each other and ourselves and have been reminded not to take any of our small daily pleasures for granted.

We always savor the holiday season as a time for

reflection as well as celebration. We have a lot to celebrate this year. Since I am trying to minimize exposure to little kids during this cold and flu season, Cameron and Murray will be with us over the holidays but not the older kids and families. Although we have gained a lot from this unplanned and unwanted journey through 2014, we do hope to have some travels next year that involve a bit more FUN. My family and I are particularly grateful that I am alive this year to celebrate the holidays and the coming year with people I love. We give thanks each day for all of you who have cheered us on during this most difficult year of our lives.

A few years ago a friend sent me an evocative Rainer Maria Rilke quote that I stuck on my corkboard so I could reread it at this time of year.

"Now let us give thanks for the new year ahead, given to us fresh, untouched, and filled with things that have never been."

With warmth and good cheer,

Kathryn

A CHRISTMAS TALE OF LOVE… AND OF GIFTS, PAST, PRESENT, AND FUTURE

Dave

December 23, 2014

Day +150.
Christmas Past.
This is a big day for me. Not because we are passing the 150th day since Kathryn's stem cell transplant, although that is a milestone in itself. No, today is the most important date in my year, the one anniversary that I never forget. It was exactly 28 years ago today that Kathryn Crawford entered my life. It was on December 23rd, 1986, on Christmas-Eve-Eve when I finally had the courage to meet this intriguing young woman on a blind

date at a dinner party in Montlake hosted by a mutual friend.

I had been "blown out the water" the previous year. My Scottish wife announced that she was dumping me... like a boring, predictable, reliable and familiar old family station wagon. She was trading me in for a younger and more exciting sporty American convertible model. I spent the next eighteen months desperately rearranging my dreams and priorities, waiting in London for months on end for a new Visa to arrive, going through my life savings, and reorganizing my life to minimize the fallout and damage and pain for my three adorable kids, Lewis (9), Wendy (7) and Roderick (5). By the summer of 1986 I was back in the USA - this harsh, unforgiving, foreign land - trying to pick up the pieces of my life in a scruffy rental house in Seattle, just off noisy Aurora Avenue, on N137th Street, walking distance from K-mart. For a Scottish country boy growing up amidst nature and solitude I might as well have been plopped down on planet Mars. Welcome to your new life, Dave. Go back to "Go." Do not collect $200...

I heard about Kathryn that summer, but didn't feel remotely ready to meet someone this intimidating. She was clearly energetic, smart, and independent. She worked as a Public Health nurse helping inmates in the King County jail stay healthy, or seeking out homeless people while they slept under the Alaskan Way viaduct, making sure that they were taking their anti-tuberculosis medications. She owned her own house... and had a second home, too – a family cabin on Vashon Island, no less. This was a woman who not only hiked and kayaked and liked to garden. That was all fine.

I could handle that. But this woman had traveled far and wide. She had a spent a summer doing rural nursing in the backwoods of the Appalachian Mountains in North Carolina. She had lived in Japan for a year. I had seen her photograph and she certainly looked cute, but what on earth would such a woman find remotely interesting in this boring, rejected, Scottish doctor with three little kids in tow? This woman had already starred in a movie, "Polka Dot Special!"... scuba diving... in a bikini... in the Micronesian islands near the Philippines... with sharks! **I kid you not!** By comparison my life had been a safe, predictable, unadventurous failure... at least that's how I felt about myself in the summer of 1986.

By December of that year I had regained a little of my self-confidence. My kids were adjusting well, I was in good physical shape, and my work was going great. I had more clinical common sense than most of my American professors. I could connect well with "regular" Americans with diabetes. I had published a couple of research papers. I had bought myself a big ol' second-hand American Ford F-150 truck with only 100,000 miles on it, which I called Henry. It only had one bench seat, which I covered with a pink sheepskin to make it comfy (and less macho-looking) for the kids, especially Wendy. So when our mutual friend asked, yet again, if I would like to come to a dinner party to meet Kathryn Crawford I decided to take the plunge. And so on Christmas-Eve-Eve, 1986, Henry and I set off for that fateful dinner party in Montlake to meet the mysterious jail-nurse-vagrant-friend-bikini-clad-scuba-diving woman...

I don't remember much about that evening. I couldn't tell you what we ate or who else was there, or even what anyone else was wearing. Kathryn was dressed rather primly, as I recall, in a smart blouse and sweater, a demure knee-length tweed skirt, dark stockings, and sensible shoes. She looked like she was dressed for a business interview... which it turned out she was! Over the next four hours Kathryn proceeded to grill me on every topic imaginable, from worldwide compassion to financial competency, from attitudes about parenting, child-rearing, politics, and spirituality, to how much discomfort I could tolerate while hiking above five thousand feet, and how much I cared about the downtrodden. There was no small talk... not even fifteen seconds of it to break the ice. She gave me a look that said,

"Okay, young man, you and I both know why we are here, so let's get going. What kind of person are you, what makes you tick, what do you want, and what do you have to offer?"

I limped home in Henry four hours later feeling exhausted and wrung out, with a vision of Kathryn's intense, penetrating, kind-yet-uncompromising eyes seared into my brain, not at all sure how the interview had gone.

As it turned out I must have said something right because I "made the cut." She agreed to talk to me again the following day and we began dating. It was a few weeks after that, in early 1987, when I felt ready to introduce Kathryn to Lewis, Wendy, and Roderick. She arrived at the house one cold January evening when the kids were almost in bed. Her entrance was memorable to say the least. I hadn't realized that to know Kathryn was also to get to know Abby. Kathryn drove a 1966 Bahama Blue Volkswagen Bug called Abby (because the license plate contained the letters ABI). Kathryn and Abby came farting along N137th Street making that unforgettable, noisy, iconic old VW Bug sound. By the time Kathryn pulled up outside our door three pairs of beady eyes were staring at her from behind the curtains, eager to catch a glimpse of this mysterious woman who had made their daddy smile and laugh for the first time in years...

My first introduction to Abby was another eye-opener. Like her owner, Abby was a unique and quirky character. Kathryn had customized her rig. With the engine in the back and only a small trunk up front Abby was way too small to accommodate the necessary gardening supplies for Kathryn's needs. Ever the problem solver Kathryn had removed the front passenger seat to create enough room to carry bales of hay, bags of compost and potting soil along with gallon pots of Huckleberry bushes and Gerbera daisies. So when Kathryn and I first went out on dates in her car I had to sit on the passenger side, but in the back seat. This had its advantages for me, however, because that way Kathryn couldn't see the sweat forming on my brow as we roared along the road. Abby, apparently, had only one speed... FAST. Abby was not going to be slowed down or encumbered by any features of comfort or safety. To be fair she did have windshield wipers that worked... after a fashion. They were able to smear grease, dirt, grime, and dead bug guts back and forth across the windshield quite effectively. Abby, however, had no working windscreen washer. But this was simply a minor inconvenience that was not going to slow Kathryn down either. As we barreled down the road in rapidly deteriorating visual conditions she calmly cranked down the window on the driver's side, letting a blast of cold air in to keep me awake, freezing, and on my toes in the back seat. Without slowing down Kathryn then reached under her seat with her left hand and brought out a squirt bottle of water. She thrust her left arm out the window, pushed it round to the front and right and proceeded to spray water from the bottle onto the front windscreen as we drove along. That vision remains with me almost thirty years later and sums up Kathryn perfectly. A problem-solver par excellence, and a woman to be reckoned with. I was hooked!

And so, although I didn't recognize it at the time, the best Christmas gift I ever got was meeting Kathryn Crawford on Christmas-Eve-Eve in 1986.

Christmas Present.

During this past year the greatest gift that I have gotten is the gift of life for Kathryn, the gift of her brand new stem cells. But miraculous and wonderful though that gift is, we now realize that it comes with a very extensive "payment plan." We will be paying with many more months and years of powerful and unpleasant drugs and their side effects in order to get the most use of that gift of life. As Kathryn mentioned in her last journal entry she is back on high dose prednisone. This time she will stay on it for longer and will taper off of it much more slowly. That feels like a body blow to Kathryn. It feels like a step backwards, and is a bitter pill to swallow, like she is not truly "getting better" yet. There are days when she struggles to keep herself feeling upbeat and positive about the life she now has to live.

It probably says a lot about me that I can quote far more lines from Tom Waits than from William Shakespeare! There is a great song called "Picture In A

Frame" from his Mule Variations album. I am sure you can listen to it on iTunes or YouTube or Spotify if you are interested. It is a sentimental song but Tom can pull it off because of his Oh-so-authentic, gravelly, cigarette-and-whisky-soaked voice, which soars in the chorus:

"I'm gonna love you till the wheels come off,
O-o-o-o-o-o-o-oh yeah..."

I played this for Kathryn recently for two reasons. Firstly, to remind her that that is exactly how I feel about her. But secondly, and much more importantly, to emphasize to her that we are not **CLOSE** to having the wheels coming off in her life. If she were a car, like Abby, and I took her to my gruff Scottish Uncle Jimmy (who ran an Auto body Car Repair business in Ayrshire when I was growing up) he would say,

"Och she's no' in bad shape, really. Her wheels are maybe a bit squeaky and shoogly right now, I'll grant you, but if we tighten up her lug-nuts and put fresh grease on her ball-bearings we'll have her running like a champ again in no time. She'll be good for another few hundred thousand miles, you mark my words."

So the handfuls of pills and central line infusions are like our lug-nut wrenches, and the mouthwashes, eye drops, and body lotions are our ball-bearing grease. With all of that plus a great attitude and a good dose of intestinal fortitude we will try to get Kathryn "running like a champ" for a few hundred thousand more miles...

Christmas Future.

My wish for the future is to have the gift of Kathryn in all of our lives for many years to come. So whether you celebrate Christmas or Hanukkah or Kwanza or the Winter Solstice... or even Seinfeld's Festivus I wish you all a Happy-Whatever-You-Choose-To-Believe-In!

I hope that 2015 will be filled with fun and adventures for all of you... and for Kathryn, too.

TRANSPLANT-YEAR-IN-REVIEW: THE SOUND BITE EDITION

Dave

December 30, 2014

Day +156: As this year comes to a close everyone from network television late night comedy shows to NPR's news magazines is putting together their year-in-review shows. Some will create "Top Ten" lists on themes of memorable events or people or songs or stories. That got me thinking. How can I best characterize this most difficult year in Kathryn's and my life? Now since this is only Day +156 you may be thinking that this should only be the Five-Months-In-Review, but in truth our long hard journey began at the very start of the year. The last "normal" social event that we had in our lives was a work-related dinner party at a colleague's house back in January where, along with several other couples, we chatted about our kids and vacation plans, politics, our favorite books and movies, all while sipping a beer or glass of wine... Two days later Kathryn got the lab test that confirmed that her blood counts were plummeting, her bone marrow was seriously malfunctioning, and that our year was going to be filled with some very different decisions than what book to read next, or where we might go on vacation.

So in the spirit of memorable lists from the Year-In-Review here is a list of sound bites and phrases that had never been uttered in the Crawford-McCulloch household in the past but have now become part of our daily lexicon:

"Dave, I'm beeping!" I have written before about our portable infusion pump and the sound it makes as it delivers a steady stream of saline and magnesium into the base of Kathryn's heart (Remember "Darth Vader In A Handbag?") When Darth Vader is getting close to being done he starts beeping, quietly at first but then with increasing volume and persistence. So whether I am napping, watching a movie, sharing a quiet moment by the fire, or folding the laundry I will hear Kathryn calling out this phrase at some point in every day.

"How are your bowels (or any number of body parts)?" I am happy to say that this is being asked less often as the year has gone on. When Kathryn was in the hospital in July she got asked this question several times a day and even after discharge at every visit to the Tan Team at SCCA during the first 100 days this was the usual opening remark by anyone entering the room. Kathryn has remained very kind and polite about this even though it is tedious and demeaning beyond belief to have the importance and meaning of your life reduced to the ritual recording of bodily functions rather than discussing the broader, more meaningful human, intellectual and spiritual thoughts and concerns that you might have.

"Clockwise or anti-clockwise?" When you feel that you have no control over your day-to-day life and that every waking minute is filled with unwelcome predetermined events that you just have to get through (counting pills, getting your infusion hooked up, making lab and clinic appointments, etc) it is nice to try to preserve at least a few situations where Kathryn gets to make a choice for herself and **decide** something! So when we set off on our daily walks around the Discovery Park Loop I will usually ask, "Clockwise or anti-clockwise?" and let Kathryn decide on the direction of our walk. If I want to be really reckless I may expand her options and add, "Do you want to do the thousand steps at the beginning or end of the walk?" or maybe even, "Want to add a mile by going down along the beach and out past the lighthouse today?" As you can imagine this will have Kathryn's head spinning with the dizzying array of exotic choices that I am tempting her with. Actually, her answer is usually determined by the time of day, when it is likely to be getting dark or start to rain, how many chores she still has to do back at the house... or whether or not she has started beeping!

"My LFTs are up again." During this year Kathryn has had to go to the lab so-o-o-o many times and for so-o-o-o many different tests that we no longer expect for everything to come back "normal." Kathryn will get messages via voice-mail, e-mail, or texts letting her know which particular lab tests are abnormal this time and by how much. She will then share that with me, who will respond with typical tenderness and compassion...

"Really? What was your tacro level?" Oh, I am

probably sharing too much of our deep intimate conversations, here, but making adjustments to keep Kathryn's fickle blood tacrolimus level in an acceptable range is another daily (or now weekly) task for us.

"Do you have your Purell and a spare battery?" Before we go out for any trip (for a walk, to the store, the clinic, the lab) we check in with each other to make sure that one or both of us has hand-sanitizer and a spare battery for the infusion pump in our pocket or purse.

"It's Coram on the phone. Do we need anything besides infusion sets and flushes?" Coram is the company used by SCCA and Group Health to deliver all the supplies for keeping the central line clean, safe, and busy. Our refrigerator has drawers full of infusion bags, saline syringes, heparin flushes, alcohol swabs...

"Oh bother, I can't have that, can I?" This frustrated phrase comes out of Kathryn's mouth whenever she lets her guard down for a second and reaches out her hand spontaneously for a piece of "forbidden food"... you know, something really toxic and dangerous like unwashed fresh fruit, a doughnut from the deli counter, a piece of sushi or smoked salmon or blue cheese or...

"Have you seen my pills?" The surfaces all over our house are decorated with piles and piles and PILES of pills. Sometimes they are still in their plastic "Mediset" sections (MORN, NOON, EVE, BED) but they may also have been moved. Some are in little bowls sitting beside a large jug of water, others might be next to tubs of yogurt. It depends on whether or not they need to be taken on an empty stomach, with food, or washed down with "two large glasses of water." You see what fascinating variety we have in our lives, these days?

"Good grief, the laundry chute is full again!" Okay, I'll admit that this particular phrase is not very exotic or unusual. I am sure that this has been uttered in your house on a regular basis, too. But unless you are living with three hyperactive teenagers or several infants with vomiting and diarrhea you are probably not doing laundry as often as we are. Everything gets used just once and then gets re-washed... cloths, dish towels, bath towels, pillow cases, bedclothes, socks, clothes, pajamas, underwear... Still in the spirit of trying to make even the most tedious of daily tasks a little more fun I have started using my "laundry time" as time to meditate on some of the deeper and more vexing philosophical questions of our time. Folding towels and color-coordinating the piles of underwear can be very soothing and contemplative. And though I am not one to brag I do believe I am making some significant scientific progress. I am close to having a plausible hypothesis for the unfathomable "Single Sock Problem." How is it that even though you always put socks into the wash in **pairs** there are always **single** socks left when you take them out of the dryer? This issue has dogged mankind for millennia, ever since we moved out of caves and decided to put socks onto our hairy, dirty feet. The answer... at least my strong working (and testable) hypothesis is... **FITTED SHEETS!** They act like deep-sea trawl nets, catching unwary socks as they spin round and round getting dizzy. They hide them in their dark flannel corners only to be discovered days later when you are making the bed with clean sheets... yet again.

"Red or white?" Unfortunately this is not the phrase that Kathryn hears when she is out for a romantic meal and the wine steward swings by our table. No, those romantic visions are a thing of the past and may not be in our future during the coming year either. No, the question, "Red or white?" means, "Which of the two central line ports do we connect the infusion to today, the red one or the white one?" Both need to be flushed with saline and heparin once a day but we try to alternate which one is used for the 2-4 hour infusion.

"I just can't eat this much food." Now this is not a phrase you will hear coming out the mouth of many Americans, I think you will agree. But Kathryn has always managed to maintain her weight within a narrow and ideal range... but is struggling to do so these days. We were warned that the ravages of the transplant regimen (the drugs, the side effects, the sleep deprivation, the exhaustion) would cause weight loss and so she needs to force-feed herself, if necessary, to keep her weight up. This is particularly problematic when she is on prednisone, which causes muscle wasting, so she needs to eat lots of extra protein. For Kathryn, food has become like more "medicine," just another pile of stuff she has to force down, even though I try to make it look and taste as appetizing as possible.

"I wonder what "regular" people are doing right now?" I am amazed at how relatively rarely Kathryn says this poignant phrase. She feels as though she has been in solitary confinement for twelve months and counting. She is going round and round in tedious circles in a dark little cul-de-sac off the main highway of life, while other "regular" people are using the highway to zoom off and do interesting things.

"I am so-o-o-o SICK of this!" This is another heartfelt statement of the obvious that Kathryn hardly ever says even though I can tell that she is thinking it multiple times every day. No amount of reading or talking about it ahead of time can prepare you for just how long and hard this journey is, but sick of it or not, we just have to keep going.

"I'd give anything to just soak in the tub with a good book and a large glass of Crown Royal!" Truthfully, I have never seen Kathryn with a **large** glass of Crown Royal in my life but it has been one of her favorite small-but-exquisite pleasures in life to end the day soaking in our claw-foot tub reading a book and sipping a small glass of Crown Royal. That too has been denied her this past year and is still a rather distant dream for her future sense of well-being and normalcy. She can't soak in the tub in case dirty water gets into her central intravenous line and causes a catastrophic blood infection. She can't see well enough to read a book by lamplight in the tub, and she can't drink any alcohol right now in case it screws up her liver function tests or messes with the various drugs she is taking...

So as this year draws to a close Kathryn and I would like to toast you all with "pretend" glasses of Crown Royal (or in my case a "pretend" glass of 17-year-old Highland Park single malt) and wish you all health and happiness, fun and laughter in the year ahead. Let's hope that it will be a better one for all of us.

THE SLOW BAD MOVIE ISN'T OVER YET

Kathryn

January 11, 2015

A few posts back Dave described our journey as a bad, slow movie. In his opinion, one of the things that makes a movie bad is that the plot is too long, boring, convoluted, or confusing. Our journey could be described as all of those. He noted that we don't even have the option of fast forwarding to see if the end makes it worth sitting through it. I am so very glad that we are the only ones who have to sit through the whole thing. So, you can all feel free to leave at any time.

As I wrote three weeks ago, I had started back on 30mg of prednisone daily but, unfortunately, that didn't control my worsening liver and mouth symptoms. This past week I saw a delightful and expert doctor, Mary

Flowers, in the Long Term Follow-up unit. She took one look at the whole picture and said I need to go up to 50mg daily. I'll be on that for at least two weeks and then the taper will be slow, so I'll be on high doses for many months. She told me that the average length of time for post-transplant patients to be immune suppressed is three years and I have no reason to believe I'll be on the short end of that so I am adjusting what I think might be possible over the next 3+ years.

This treatment change felt like a body blow to Dave and me since it extends the time that I will not feel well and increases the chances of long-term consequences from the drug. It also means I probably can't get my central line out any time soon since I may need more IVs at home to prevent infections. Feeling weak, jittery, under-slept, and like I can't think are the worst effects for me. And nobody really loves the chipmunk look. I do hope for days of basic physical comfort in the future.

In spite of this setback, we try to find a bit of fun or humor in every day and appreciate the little everyday pleasures in life. Dave has been a stalwart and good-humored companion throughout all of this but I don't think we are laughing enough. Shortly before my transplant I visited the mother of an old friend. Her name is Velda, she is 92, and was just finishing a master's degree. Two months before her second husband had died. I asked her about what she had learned about dealing with grief during her long life. She said she had three rules:

1)Do things you don't want to do, meaning get out of the house even if you don't really feel like it.

2)See people you don't want to see, meaning be sociable even when you may not feel like it so that you don't become too isolated.
3)Laugh at least once every day.

I have really taken Velda's rules to heart and feel like they apply in various difficult life circumstances.

Please feel free to send along anything you find good for a laugh. Someone sent me a link to one-star Yelp reviews of National Parks that was hilarious. I love that the days are getting longer and my hellebores under the witch hazel are beginning to bloom. I have some wonderful plants that come back year after year from my friends at the Group Health Rainier Valley Medical Center where I used to work. We have terrific winter pots that Gabriella planted and their beauty is soothing to me.

Dave and I are still hoping to have a building permit and to begin building our house on Vashon this coming summer. We are looking forward to all our kids and grandkids being around for some island camping and beach time.

Addendum: I hadn't finished typing this when I went to bed last night. I woke at midnight with a fast, irregular pulse and felt a bit short of breath, sort of like the night in October. We got to the Emergency Room at Virginia Mason about 1 a.m. and my pulse had settled enough that they put me back on the heart medication I stopped a week ago and I got to go home. Just when I think maybe we can begin to shift our life focus **away** from my body, we get jerked back to some new or recurrent problem. All we can do is take in the news, recalibrate our expectations, and move back to a place of centeredness about how to move forward. Thanks to all of you who help us maintain our fortitude as I work toward healing and brighter days.

Best wishes to all of you for 2015. May the New Year bring what you wish for most.

Love,
Kathryn

PROVERBS AND PLATITUDES

Dave

January 17, 2015

Day +175: I don't know if you have noticed but proverbs are very popular these days. Everywhere you go there are inspirational sayings that are meant to make you think, "Wow, that is so deep!" or pieces of supposedly ancient wisdom that stop you for a moment to say, "Huh? I'd never thought of it like that!" You can see them on the sides of buses helping to advertise beer. They are a staple of Hallmark greetings cards. And if you walk into the palatial office of your company's CEO you're sure to find one framed and hanging on the wall behind his or her desk. It is there to tell you, "I'm not just an overpaid ass, I used to be a lowly mortal like you. This piece of wisdom has inspired me to greatness. This proverb encapsulates my personal "True North." (Feel free to gag before you leave his or her office.) And you can buy entire books of inspirational phrases and proverbs, these days. They are usually overpriced, with puffy padded covers, and printed on expensive paper with one inspirational saying on each page so that when you are feeling down you can flip to any random page and go, "Wow, that is so true! Now the rest of my day and life will go a lot better!"

Now don't get me wrong, I like a nice pithy piece of wisdom just as much as the next guy but the slightly cynical part of me has noticed that they can be a bit self-righteous and preachy and that some of what they say is just a tired platitude. But authors in the new "Proverb Industry" have several different ways to make you more inclined to believe them. Now I may be wrong but I doubt whether Confucius, back in 500BC, was secretly hoping that his inscrutable thoughts would help to sell Lite beer and pickup trucks in America 2,500 years later! And have you noticed how many sayings are attributed to Winston Churchill, Mark Twain, or Oscar Wilde? Now I grant you those were three very witty, smart people but I think authors in the "Proverb Industry" attach the names of one of those famous guys to a pithy saying just to make the reader more likely to believe it and be more impressed. Sometimes it is easy to tell when this tactic is fake, though:

"When it's two outs in the bottom of the ninth and you're up to bat you need to look straight ahead, take a deep breath, and make a good solid swing."

Oscar Wilde

That one just doesn't ring true to me. You'll

notice that any ancient wisdom involving rainbows or pots of gold will be said to be ***Irish***. And if the saying is particularly confusing or obscure and you are about to roll your eyes and dismiss it as nonsense they will put ***Ancient Chinese Saying*** after it to make you think twice. Try this one for example:

"The rays of the morning sun are like the feathers of a flightless bird walking backwards through the forest."
Ancient Chinese Saying

Now before you start doing mental gymnastics trying to parse a deeper meaning out of that inscrutable oriental gem I should tell you that I just made all that up by putting a bunch of random things together into a convoluted sentence! The point is that you are much more likely to try to think deeply about it if you think it is an ***Ancient Chinese Saying*** rather than ***One Of Dave's Smart-Aleck Remarks***.

So what has all this rambling got to do with Kathryn and me and our uncertain journey, you might ask? Well, at work one of the administrative support people in our department has started writing inspirational sayings or proverbs on a blackboard near her desk as something fun to entertain her colleagues with, to stimulate conversation, and improve staff morale. Her name is Rena Ortigoza. She is a lovely person, very caring, always perky and upbeat, and I very much enjoy working with her. I applaud the idea of her "Inspirational Blackboard." I confess that I look forward to seeing what will show up there next although I have to say they more often make me laugh and roll my eyes than perhaps they should. The one she posted last week made me both scoff and reflect. It read:

"If you just keep putting one foot in front of the next, eventually you will look back and realize... that you have climbed a mountain."

African Proverb

That one really made me gag! African proverb? Really? I don't think of Africans as people who spend a lot of time climbing mountains, although, come to think of it, that might be the only place left to go to escape from Ebola, corrupt dictators, or marauding bands of murderous lunatics like Boko Haram. But even if it is not an African proverb I just don't get this fascination that the "Proverb Industry" has with the metaphor about climbing mountains. Why is that such a good idea? By the time you have climbed a really big mountain you are probably out of breath, soaking wet, and freezing cold. Chances are you are completely sick of eating freeze-dried protein bars washed down with melted snow or distilled urine. And now what are you going to do, now that you are at the top of your mountain? If you have any sense and aren't hallucinating from anoxia or passing out from hypothermia then you will gingerly trudge back down the mountain as quickly as you can without breaking your neck and look for a nice sunny valley with a hammock, a pile of good books to read, and a large pitcher of lemonade or beer to drink.

So for the journey that Kathryn and I are on I don't like the mountain metaphor too much. I prefer to think that our destination might be filled with hammocks, sunshine, good books and beer! Besides, that so-called ***African Proverb*** seems pretty stupid to me in a lot of ways. I can think of a few more accurate ways to complete that sentence:

"If you just keep putting one foot in front of the next, eventually you will look back and realize... that you have been walking around and around in circles!"

Anonymous Pessimist

In some ways that "proverb" resonates better with how Kathryn and I are feeling right now. We are back on high dose prednisone... **again**... have low magnesium...**again**... and had another episode of atrial fibrillation...**again**. Neither of us wants to keep going around and around in these circles too much longer.

Here is another alternative ending that came to my mind:

"If you just keep putting one foot in front of the next, eventually you will look back and realize... that you are in the bad part of town, you are completely lost, it is 1am, and the battery in your cell phone just died!"

Grumpy Scottish Cynic

There are days when that is how this uncertain journey feels to me.

But not often! My default state-of-being is optimistic and ready to take on a new challenge with enthusiasm. So here we are on **Day +175**. We have another appointment next week with the energetic and knowledgeable chief physician at the stem cell transplant Long Term Follow-up Unit, the incomparable Mary Flowers. She has made it clear, based on what she sees after talking to Kathryn, examining her, and looking at

Kathryn's labs, that she will confidently make an adjustment and set us off putting one foot in front of the next in a new direction.

I plan to bring a sturdy pair of walking shoes with me to the appointment, along with plenty of water and protein bars, a spare battery... and maybe a compass.

OF MICE AND MEN... AND WOMEN
PART ONE

Dave

January 25, 2015

Day +183: I've been thinking a lot about mice recently. Let me tell you two mice stories. One of them is based on observations that I've made in the past two weeks. The second is some reflections on a poem written over two hundred years ago. I'll then try to connect them to how Kathryn and I are feeling as we start this New Year.

Two weeks ago

We have had a bad start to this year. Within a few weeks of stopping prednisone Kathryn's liver enzymes began to rise and painful sores began to reappear in her mouth. Even when she was started back on a "moderate" dose of prednisone (0.5mg/kg) things didn't improve. Since she has been on a therapeutic dose of tacrolimus during all this time (with blood levels checked weekly to make sure) her doctors were at a loss what to do next so they sent her back to the Seattle Cancer Care Alliance (SCCA) to see Dr. Mary Flowers, a brilliant physician who hails from Brazil and now leads the Long Term Follow-up Unit (LTFU).

We got there in plenty of time and began to reminisce about the familiar surroundings and routines that had been our daily routine for the first 100 days after Kathryn's stem cell transplantation. Hand sanitizers and masks were everywhere along with "free" bottles of filtered water at every check-in desk, nice artwork on the walls, and panoramic views of the Sea Planes taking off and landing on Lake Union. We quietly observed the other patients and families sitting around in groups expressing varying degrees of optimism, sadness, and suffering in their eyes, words, and body language. And then we heard the familiar disembodied voice announce,

"Richardson, room 11, Takayama, room 16, Crawford, room 27..."

A friendly-but-unfamiliar Medical Assistant came in first, followed by another new Nurse Practitioner. They were very thorough and detailed as they asked questions, inspected Kathryn's skin, mouth and eyes, and then left to go get the famous Dr. Flowers. We must have waited forty-five minutes, chatting and sighing wearily, before the door burst open and in came Mary Flowers followed by a small entourage of Brazilian research fellows, support staff and nurses. My immediate impression of Dr. Flowers was that she was a bustling, energetic mouse escorting her little family into the room. I don't mean that to sound pejorative in the least. She fizzed with intelligence and energy and immediately commanded the room. But she was tiny, with straight brown hair surrounding a small round face. She had a sharp nose and intense eyes that sparkled with inquisitiveness and good humor from behind her large round glasses.

"So sorry I'm late but you are s-o-o-o interesting! I wanted to read a-a-a-all of your chart notes so that I understand exactly what is going on."

She whirled around and brought her face close to Kathryn's as if they were the only two people in the room.

"So tell me, what bothers you the most... right now... what you worry about the most?"

Kathryn explained that her eyes were still her biggest problem. She was also worried about her bones disappearing altogether if she had to stay on high dose prednisone for months on end. She wanted to understand why her mouth and liver were getting worse, and what, if anything, could be done about these issues. For the next thirty minutes the professorial mouse scurried around the room asking questions, giving explanations, and engaging everyone in the room, including me.

"I hear you a doctor. What kind? Where you from? You have an accent. I have accent, too. I came from Brazil but I've been here a lo-o-ong time. How **you** think Kathryn is doing?"

Although animated and quick to respond, Dr. Flowers listened very carefully and answered every one of Kathryn's long list of questions before she came up with a new plan.

"You have chronic GVHD, right? It's clear. We know that. This means you gonna need to be on immunosuppressive drugs for 2-3 years... Maybe less, maybe more, we don't know. But you look good! You strong, you exercising... a LOT. You eat healthy. So you're Grade 1 chronic GVHD. You should do very well but this is what we know. You respond to prednisone very well, so that's good, but when we take you off again the GVHD comes back so that's not good. The tacrolimus can't keep the GVHD in check on its own. But maybe if we switch you from tacrolimus to **sirolimus** then we can control your GVHD on much lower doses of prednisone. That would be good. It will take time for your new stem cells to settle down so we all need to be patient, okay? What other questions you have?"

So now we have a better understanding of what is going on and what to expect. Kathryn is tapering off her tacrolimus in the next two weeks and getting established on an effective dose of sirolimus. Sirolimus is a cousin of tacrolimus, another Roman Centurion to protect Kathryn's body from the over-zealous new stem cells cruising around inside of her. Sirolimus is younger (i.e. a newer drug) than tacrolimus and has a different personality (or side effects!). Kathryn might notice less trembling in her hands, less burning in her feet, and her magnesium levels might come back up. Those would all be welcome changes for us! But sirolimus can cause a host of other side effects. Her cholesterol and triglycerides (another fat in the blood) may go up and might cause her platelets and white cells to go down a bit so we will need to continue to be vigilant and do weekly blood tests.

But as the bustling professorial mouse left us with beaming smiles and vigorous handshakes (followed by ritual hand-sanitizing by everyone in the room, of course!) we both felt a lot more optimism. There are no guarantees, of course, but we feel sure that we have a new person on our team - someone who seems very competent, compassionate and caring.

OF MICE AND MEN... AND WOMEN
PART TWO

Dave

January 25, 2015

Over Two Hundred Years Ago

Day +183: January 25th is a very propitious day for me. Not only is this Day +183, exactly six months after the Jersey cells were infused into Kathryn's body. January 25th, 1759, is also the birthdate of Scotland's most famous poet, Robert Burns. Burns is much admired around the world, and there will be tens of thousands of parties (usually called ***Burns Suppers***) going on in dozens of countries tonight, celebrating his life and work. Burns came from a lowly background and grew up in a tiny farm cottage in the village of Alloway, in Ayrshire. He was a romantic, a contemporary of Keats, Wordsworth, and Sir Walter Scott. Burns fell in love frequently and wrote marvelous love songs that have been set to music. He was an intelligent young man, had a sharp wit, and was a true man-of-the-people. He detested pomposity and deceit of all sorts, especially the hypocrisy displayed by bureaucrats and religious leaders.

I spent my formative teen years in a house less than half a mile from Burns Cottage in Alloway. I fell in love just as often as Burns did (although with much less success!) I walked the same fields, and felt the same cold Scottish rain on my face. I have sung many of his wonderful songs while standing around the piano as my dad or brother played the tunes:

O My Love Is Like A Red, Red Rose.
Ye Banks And Braes Of Bonny Doon.
Flow Gently Sweet Afton.
and many more...

One of Robert Burns' most famous poems is called, ***"To A Mouse."*** It is a little masterpiece written in eight verses. The seventh verse contains one of the most frequently quoted (and even more frequently **mis**-quoted!) lines in literature. I know the poem by heart and can recite it, when invited, at parties and other gatherings. But I have noticed that when I recite it to an American audience their eyes quickly glaze over and a vacant smile spreads over their faces. They have stopped trying to understand what the poem is saying. Instead they are letting the strange, evocative, guttural sounds of the Scottish dialect, with its "Ochs" and "Grrrs" and "Sprrrrachchles" wash over them like pleasant auditory wallpaper! I have noticed the same thing, sometimes, when I am seeing diabetic patients and their families during medical appointments. When I have listened to their concerns, evaluated the situation, and am trying to offer a helpful medical treatment plan for them to consider I can see their eyes glazing over.

"Oh just keep talking Dr. McCulloch, I could listen to that lovely brogue all day."

Hmmm, as a caring physician that is problematic for me. I want the people I see to leave feeling listened to, comforted, and with a plan that they helped develop, believe in, and are enthusiastic about putting into action! It is the content of the words that I want them to appreciate, not just how nice it all sounds as it reverberates off the examination room walls.

So while I love the bold, alliterative musicality of the Scottish language I want to set up, explain, and translate this lovely poem for you before I give it to you in its original form. For any of you who hate poetry please feel free to skip the rest of this journal entry. However, I know that several of the people who are following Kathryn's journey appreciate reading and in some cases writing their own poetry.

This poem was written in 1785, when Burns was aged 26 and working as a farm laborer in the South West of Scotland. The full title of the poem is ***"To A Mouse, on turning her up in her nest with the plough, November 1785."*** Imagine a cold autumn afternoon. After a weary day following along behind the horse pulling the plough blade through the soil young Robert's mind is wandering. The field has already been harvested. The wheat, corn, or barley has long ago been sent to the mill. His job is to turn over all the dead plant stalks and root balls into the soil so that they can decay into compost to make the field ready to be planted with fresh seed the following Spring. No doubt Robert is thinking about girls, or about what the future might hold for him if he left rural Ayrshire to get a job in a big city like Edinburgh.

And then the blade of the plough cuts through the nest of a little field mouse and the terrified creature starts scurrying back and forth in front of him. Field mice are vermin, are they not? They eat the crops of oats and barley? They spread disease? He should kill it by stamping his foot on it or whacking it with a spade, right? Instead Burns is devastated at the unwitting carnage he has created. He decides to write a poem of apology to the mouse and in so doing has created a beautiful piece of writing that is a meaningful commentary on the human condition that still resonates over two hundred years later. Let me give you a rough translation.

TO A MOUSE
By Robert Burns

Little, glossy-coated timorous creature,
O, what a panic is in your breast!
You need not run away so quickly,
With rushing and scurrying!
I'm not going to run and chase you,
With my murdering spade!

I am truly sorry that man's dominion
Has broken Nature's social union,
And justifies that ill opinion,
Which makes you startle
At me, your poor, earth-born companion,
And fellow mortal!

I have no doubt that you sometimes steal,
But what of it? Poor creature, you've got to live!
The occasional ear of corn among twenty-four stacks
Is a small request;
I'll do just fine with the remainder,
And never miss it!

Your little house now lies in ruins!
Its feeble walls are scattered by the wind!
And there is no coarse grass left for you to build a
new one,
And bleak December's wind is growing
Both bitter and keen!

You saw the fields lying bare and empty,
And weary winter coming fast,
And cozy here, beneath the blast,
You thought to dwell,
Till crash! The cruel plow cut through
The walls of your house.

That little heap of leaves and stubble,
Has cost you many a weary nibble!
Now you have been turned out for all your trouble,
Without a house or shelter,
To suffer winter's wet rain and sleet,
And bitter frost!

But Little Mouse, you are not alone,
In proving that foresight may be in vain,
The best laid schemes of mice and men
Often fall apart,
And leave us nothing but grief and pain,

Instead of the joy we expected!

Still, you are blessed, compared with me!
You are only concerned with the present
But oh! I cast my eye backwards
On dismal events in my past!
And although I cannot see the future,
I can guess and fear what lies ahead.

Now here is the poem in the original Scottish dialect:

On turning her up in her nest with the plough, November, 1785
By Robert Burns

Wee sleekit, cow'rin, tim'rous beastie,
O, what a panic's in thy breastie!
Thou need na start awa sae hasty,
Wi bickering brattle!
I wad be laith to rin and chase thee,
Wi murdering pattle!

I'm truly sorry man's dominion
Has broken Nature's social union,
An justifies that ill opinion,
Which makes thee startle
At me, thy poor, earth-born companion,
An fellow mortal!

I doubt na, whyles but thou may thieve;
What then? poor beastie, thou maun live!
A daimen icker in a thrave

'S a sma request;
I'll get a blessin wi the lave,
An never miss't!

Thy wee-bit housie, too, in ruin!
Its silly wa's the win's are strewin!
An naething, now, to big a new ane,
O foggage green!
An bleak December's win's ensuin,
Baith snell an keen!

Thou saw the fields laid bare an waste,
An weary winter comin fast,
An cozie here, beneath the blast,
Thou thought to dwell,
Till crash! the cruel coulter past
Out thro thy cell.

That wee bit heap o leaves and stibble,
Has cost thee monie a' weary nibble!
Now thou's turn'd out, for a thy trouble,
But house or hald,
To thole the winter's sleety dribble,
An cranreuch cauld!

But Mousie, thou art no thy lane,
In proving foresight may be vain:
The best-laid schemes o mice an men
Gang aft agley,
An lea'e us nought but grief an pain,
For promis'd joy!

Still thou are blest compar'd wi me!

The present only toucheth thee;
But och! I backward cast my e'e,
On prospects drear!
An forward, tho I canna see,
I guess an fear!

I always think of Kathryn when I read this poem. Not that I identify her with the mouse! Far from it. That is no "cow'rin, tim'rous beastie" who lies beside me in bed at night! No, Kathryn is much more like the ploughman, like the young Robert Burns. Kathryn cares deeply about the small, the downtrodden, the disadvantaged creatures of the world, be they human or from some other species. Part of Kathryn's frustration as she keeps dealing with new bodily aggravations and health problems is that she still feels like she has so much more she would like to do to help others. She is impatient to get better so that she can take on new challenges and do more good in the world.

I love the way that Burns ends the poem. There is no sugary, artificial optimism in that last verse. He simply states the eternal human truth that none of us knows what the future holds, and if we are honest with ourselves we must feel some apprehension about what lies ahead.

This does not mean that we should not stay optimistic, however! There is much that we can control that will improve what is in store for us in the future. So how am I feeling on **Day +183?** I feel very optimistic that some combination of drugs will help Kathryn's new immune system to "settle down" and learn to live in harmony with her body. I am confident that she and I will do everything in our powers to maximize the chances of a good outcome and a happy future. There are all sorts of exciting things that we are scheming about and plan to do in the future. But it serves us all well to remember the often-quoted (or misquoted) lines of Robert Burns:

The best-laid schemes o mice an men
Gang aft agley,
An lea'e us nought but grief an pain,
For promis'd joy!

Here's hoping for less grief and pain in the months and years to come!

BROKEN HEARTS AND DIRTY WINDOWS

Dave

February 18, 2015

Day +207: Kathryn sat on my lap yesterday evening and bawled her eyes out as we listened to John Prine singing to us from across the room. John Prine is a wonderful storyteller from Kathryn and my generation. He writes about the eternal themes of love, war, and heartbreak, and sings with great tenderness and authenticity. If you are interested you should check out his album, "Souvenirs" on iTunes, or YouTube, or Spotify, or wherever you go for music these days. The line that set Kathryn off was,

> ***Broken hearts and dirty windows,***
> ***Make life difficult to see...***

Through tears of frustration she said, "When I

woke up this morning I wanted to go to work. I didn't want to have to spend the day going to the lab for more blood tests and an EKG and then have to drive to Federal Way to visit yet another goddamned wig shop."

I guess for Kathryn the line might be,

Relentless GVHD and high dose prednisone,
Make life difficult to see...

I don't have any major news to share, really, as we pass Day +200. Here's the abbreviated medical update.

Kathryn is now off tacrolimus and is on a stable dose of sirolimus. This, along with prednisone has tamped down her LFTs back to near normal and there are no signs of GVH in her mouth, skin or elsewhere for the moment. The prednisone is being tapered more slowly this time. We have a follow up appointment with Dr. Mary Flowers in a couple of weeks so it will be good to get her perspective on Kathryn's progress at that time.

We have seen a couple of people to get advice on how best to protect Kathryn's bones from the ravages of prednisone. It is complicated, and not at all clear whether she should take estrogen or a bisphosphonate or something else and, if so, starting when and for how long. We'll try to come to a good decision about that in the next few weeks.

Kathryn's heart continues to misbehave from time to time. She gets episodes where her heart rhythm is irregular and she feels lightheaded. Her heart rate never gets too fast, however, since she is taking a drug called metoprolol that holds it back but it is a bit unsettling having the rhythm change at random times during the day. She is going to wear a continuous electrical monitor of her heart for a few days to give the cardiologist more data to look at before we decide if something new needs to be done for that. Both sirolimus and prednisone can cause heart arrhythmias among their side effects. Since Kathryn still has her Hickman central line in place, part of me wonders if having a Teflon tube tickling the inside of her right atrium might be contributing to the heart's irritability, too. We may ask the cardiologist about that once the continuous monitor results are back.

Otherwise we continue our tedious-but-time-consuming routines of pills, infusions, careful food prep, walks and stair trudging...

John Prine has another lovely song called, "Hello In There," about the cruel reality of growing old and becoming invisible and ignored by younger people.

So if you're walking down the street sometime,
And spot some hollow, ancient eyes,
Please don't just pass 'em by and stare,
As if you didn't care,
Say, hello in there,
Hello...

Right now Kathryn and I are hoping we'll be lucky enough to live long enough to suffer that indignity some day, too!

TEDIOUS DRUG DETAIL UPDATE

Dave

February 22, 2015

Day +211: As Spring is bursting into action here in Seattle it has got me reflecting on Spring days from my past and the numerous connections that I have had between Scotland and the USA over the years. I will write about that in a separate post ("Spring Is Sprung") but even though it is dull reading for most people I want to record here what Kathryn's current drug regimen looks like on Day +211:

Prednisone 40mg and 5mg on alternate days (part of a very slow taper) - for systemic GVHD treatment

Sirolimus 2mg or 1.5mg daily depending on weekly lab tests - for systemic GVHD treatment

Dexamethasone elixir 0.1mg/ml, mouthwash for

four minutes four times a day - for local mouth GVH

Clotrimazole troches 10mg four times a day - to help prevent yeast infection in the mouth that can happen because of the Dexamethasone

Cyclosporine eye drops 0.05% twice daily in each eye - for local eye GVHD treatment

Trimethoprim sulfa DS once daily - prophylaxis against bacterial infection that can happen because of the immunosuppression that KC is on

Acyclovir 800mg twice daily - prophylaxis against viral infection that can happen because of the immunosuppression that KC is on

Metoprolol XL 25mg daily to slow down Kathryn's heart rate if she flips in and out of Atrial Fibrillation

Ursadiol 300mg twice daily - prophylaxis against GVHD occurring in the liver

Pravastatin 10mg once daily - to protect against heart attacks and to lower the high cholesterol caused by sirolimus

Potassium phosphate 250mg twice daily

Magnesium oxide 800mg twice daily

Magnesium plus protein 133mg, six tablets daily

Magnesium chloride infusion 40mg over two hours by IV infusion pump

Sodium fluoride gel once daily on the teeth at bedtime - to protect the teeth, which are more vulnerable to damage due to GVHD-dry mouth

Multivitamin one daily - since all Americans need to eat multivitamins, right?

Calcium citrate 1200mg daily - to help protect the bones from disappearing because of high dose prednisone

Vitamin D 1000mg daily - to help protect the

bones from disappearing because of high dose prednisone

(Tacrolimus was stopped about two weeks ago)

(Beclomethasone in corn oil was stopped over a month ago since it is no longer needed to prevent gut GVHD since she is back on high dose prednisone)

(KC decided to stop Pantoprazole recently because acid reflux and GI discomfort are not a problem right now)

I am struck with what a long list this is for someone who has taken such great care of her health over the past 61 years. However, we both need to just get over how unfair it all seems. This ever-changing cocktail of drugs is trying to help tamp down the vigorous GVH disease being mounted by the new stem cells that have been settling in over the past 211 days, but it is also treating the real or potential side effects from other drugs on the list.

I think Kathryn will give an update of how she is feeling about things later today.

SPRING IS SPRUNG!

Dave: February 22, 2015

Day +211: As Kathryn and I trudged around the Loop Trail this morning comparing notes on which of our various joints and muscles hurt the most I was struck with how vigorously signs of spring are asserting themselves in a riotous palette of green. The leaves of the Indian plum are sturdy and upright. Stinging nettles are pushing through the brown decaying autumn leaves, and a flowering currant is already showing off its dangling pink blossoms. All of these are plants that were very familiar to me growing up in rural Scotland.

Like most country boys, nettles played a big role in my life! The theory circulating among all the boys in the school playground was that nettles were at their stingiest and deadliest when they first emerged from the ground and were about a foot tall with vigorous new spring growth on them. However, if you were brave enough and grabbed the nettle near the top and crushed it in your fist as you ripped it off from the rest of the plant then you wouldn't get stung! If you DID get stung it was because you had been too tentative or just weren't brave enough to crush it hard enough. I have vivid memories of seeing several small boys walking around the playground shaking their welt-covered hands in the air and trying to hold back the tears.

Even as a seven-year old boy growing up in a fishing village in the Southwest of Scotland I was strongly influenced by the romance and excitement of America. When we got our first ever small black and white television I was only allowed to watch half an hour every day and only if I had done all of my homework, of course, so I had to be ve-e-e-ery selective about what I watched. I had three absolute favorites: the cartoon of Popeye-the-sailor-man slurping up cans of spinach through his pipe, The Lone Ranger riding into town with his deferential Indian side-kick, Tonto, and Bonanza, where the Cartwright family cast their wisdom, integrity, bravery, and machismo over a vast wilderness of prairies and mesas and an anonymous and mysterious forest called the Ponderosa. I was so obsessed with all things American that I pleaded to get a Lone Ranger outfit for Christmas one year. When it came it was totally perfect. It had a jacket and pants in matching pale blue and white pinstripes. Sewn into the bottom of the pants was a black felt extension that covered your shoes so that it looked like you were wearing authentic cowboy boots with the pinstripe pants tucked inside. The outfit came, of course, with a belt, two holsters, and a pair of six-shooters: Peacemaker Colts which held rolls of "caps" that made satisfyingly loud bangs when you pulled the trigger and gave off a pleasant smell of gunpowder smoke. For those of you unfamiliar with "cap guns" the "caps" were small collections of gunpowder, about a quarter inch in diameter, that were contained in a thin roll of paper (like a roll of stamps or Scotch tape). Every time you pulled the trigger the roll moved to place a new spot of gunpowder between the hammer and plate of the gun so that you had a plentiful supply of satisfying explosive sounds and "cordite" smells to accompany you on your adventures.

It all felt totally authentic to my seven-year-old imagination. The illusion was only broken (and only slightly) if you fired the guns too often in a row because that caused a long trail of spent cap paper to curl out of the top of the gun. That never happened to The Lone Ranger! But hey, you could always just rip off the spent cap paper and toss it aside to re-establish the sense of complete authenticity. Besides, I was wearing my black Lone Ranger mask so no one in our tiny village had ANY idea who this dangerous and mysterious stranger was who sauntered down the high street twirling his six-shooter on his index fingers with stunning dexterity! They just knew that they had better stay away from him...

I cheerfully took selected aspects of my three favorite shows and merged them into my own fantasy adventures. Popeye had by far the strongest and coolest American accent so I learned to mimic Popeye to amuse my friends as we hid behind damp Scottish sycamore trees in the little wood behind my house, which, in our imagination, was the vast, dangerous, and unknown Ponderosa forest. As the leader of our posse of three (since I was the only one with a Lone Ranger outfit) I would cast my worldly and experienced seven-year-old eye across the damp verdant forest floor before reciting one of Popeye's more famous sayings in as strong an American accent as I could muster:

"Spring is sprung,
The grass is rizz,
I wonders where da boidies is?
Hark, da boid is on da wing!
Don't be silly, that's absoid,
Da wing is on da boid!"

This of course would have my two pals and fellow gunslingers rolling on the ground howling with laughter.

I wore that Lone Ranger outfit for so many years that not only did the seam on the pant butt rip apart but the black felt extensions no longer covered my shoes but instead stuck out like black triangular flags half way up my shins!

You may be wondering what any of this has to do with Kathryn's progress... and the answer is, nothing at all really, except that on this sunny spring day here on Day +211 we felt able to chat and reminisce about topics other than an inventory of symptoms, drug doses and upcoming medical appointments.

That Lone Ranger outfit and awesome cap gun reminds me of another vivid childhood memory. My older brother, Bill, was bored one Saturday morning when I got back from the tiny post office/sweetie shop/ toy store after spending my pocket money on two fresh rolls of "caps."

"Hey David, want me to show you a much better way to use your caps?"

Bill was five years older than me and so clearly had much more sophisticated and exciting ideas for fun. I dutifully handed over one precious roll of caps and followed Bill to the garden shed. He rummaged around and found two large bolts, each about six inches long and about half an inch in diameter. He then found a large nut that fit the thread on the end of both bolts. He screwed the nut just a few turns onto one of the bolts. This left a hollow where the nut came off the end of the bolt. With a pair of scissors Bill then carefully cut around several dozen of the caps and crammed them into this hollow. When it was almost full he then screwed the other bolt onto the nut until it was firm and tight. Bill smiled with satisfaction and anticipation, his pleasure heightened by the look of bafflement on my face...

There was a large wall at the bottom of our garden that rose eight feet above the street below. Across the street was a row of cottages including one belonging to Mrs. McCallum, the grades 1 and 2 elementary teacher at our school. Bill waited until the street was empty before saying,

"Watch this!"

He lobbed the contraption high into the air - two heavy six-inch long bolts attached firmly together with a large nut containing tightly packed explosives in between the ends of the bolts. Just as it twirled high above us and began to fall back to the ground the front door to Mrs. McCallum's cottage began to open. Bill gasped in horror. The bolts tumbled slowly, as if in slow motion, landing firmly on one end. With an enormous BANG the bolts blew apart, one of them whistling past our heads, the other one smashing into the wall of Mrs. McCallum's cottage, luckily missing the door, the window, or Mrs. McCallum, who screamed and shut the door again. Bill and I ran off back through the garden and off into the Ponderosa where we hid out for an hour or two to avoid being captured by whatever posse would soon be sent off to bring us to justice. We wouldn't have been hard to find, mind you, laughing and squealing with delight. Bill's legendary heroism went up a few more notches in my estimation that day. Spring days don't get much better than that for a seven-year-old boy.

Little did I know then that I would end up spending most of my life living in that mysterious place called America, or that I would have many different kinds of adventures there! Neither Kathryn nor I are relishing the particular "adventure" we are in the middle of right now but we are certainly trying to make the best of it and I feel confident that we will have many more exciting adventures ahead of us. Our walk this morning reminded us that we have gone through four complete seasons in these familiar woods since we began our almost daily therapeutic walks in Discovery Park. Let's hope that the optimism of new growth, new life, and fresh starts transfers itself to us as we start the second year of this journey.

THE RUSH TO NORMAL

Kathryn

February 23, 2015

This week a friend sent me a New York Times opinion piece titled, ***The Trauma of Being Alive, by Mark Epstein***. It resonated with how I'm feeling at this point in my recovery. Although the article has a focus on the author's mother, the main ideas seem applicable to everyone. He writes about three things that seem important to me about traumas big and small - the desire to get past it and rush back to "normal," the willingness to "lean in" to the trauma if we want to heal, and the importance of experiencing the depth of our own suffering if we want to be truly open to the suffering of others. All of these seem like important things to consider if we want to be healthy and whole and compassionate.

(A side note about "leaning in." I am casually

following the national conversation about women in the workplace/leadership and have read Sheryl Sandberg's book, **Lean In**. Epstein uses that term here and it seems like it's appearing here and there as a new verb meaning to take things head on.)

What I notice in myself at this point is my own rush to get back to something that feels sort of "normal." Maybe it doesn't really even count as a rush though since I am now a full year into being unwell. As most of you know, this constricted kind of life is really testing my patience. Some days I feel like I may never get off the prednisone taper treadmill. Maybe I will find patience I never knew I could muster because I am still quite a ways off from feeling back to any kind of "normal." I was told to allow a full year for recovery after transplant but it feels SO long, and I'm just passing half way.

Epstein also writes that if we try not to feel the full impact of our trauma we deprive ourselves of its truth. For some reason I am naturally inclined to face my struggles head on. This, despite the fact that I was raised to pretend to others, and maybe even to myself, that everything was always great. I figured out by the time I was about 20 that this wasn't a healthy way to live. It doesn't work to pretend I am never frustrated, discouraged, angry or sad. The best way for me to get through hard times is to let myself feel all the ups and downs. I don't have it all together in my life and I never will. I agree with Epstein that going through hard times ourselves helps us more deeply understand the suffering of others, a gift indeed.

Epstein suggests that trauma is not just the result of major disasters but is a part of everyone's life at some point. I loved his line, "An undercurrent of trauma runs through ordinary life, shot through as it is with the poignancy of impermanence." Dave and my experience has focused us on the evanescent aspects of life. The uncertainty about what the coming year may bring is still the hardest part.

As for my recovery, my prednisone taper continues at a very slow pace. My liver numbers, the most easily measured indication of GVHD, are slowly coming down. I still have prednisone side effects and my eyes remain my biggest problem day to day. My cardiac monitor came today so I will soon be hooked up to that. I am hoping for some benign explanation for my heart irregularities since I'm trying to get **rid** of specialists, not add them. My central line is still in place and I get a daily magnesium infusion at home. I am still walking and doing weights and stairs each day with hopes of regaining strength and muscle, if not hair (!) One of the hardest things about this recovery is that many of the required activities are boring, and my tolerance for boredom has always been **low**.

As one reader implied in a Caring Bridge comment, our experience has made it clear to her that allogeneic stem cell transplants are not yet to the point of being "routine" care for blood cancers. Before I agreed to proceed with a transplant I tried to find people who had been through the experience. When someone told me they knew of someone who had had a transplant I could tell how close they were to the experience by the way they described it. The people who were close to it were quite solemn. I now know that the people who cheerily suggested that I just go get a transplant really had no idea what is involved. Of the six people I talked to, four have some residual effects but are doing well, and two have died. For many transplant patients, they are trading what might be a "cure" for a disease that will definitely kill them for a new and unpredictable disease (GVHD) that only might kill them. Although I feel like my old life is **gone**, I remain hopeful that eventually I will be able to do some of the things that are most important to me.

Many thanks to those of you who have sent me laughs of various kinds--laughing really does help. Having Cameron around home means having ready access to suggestions for stand-up comedians to watch. I had a little laugh when Dave and I recently spent a night in a hotel. There was a full-length mirror in the room and I was shocked to see what my naked body now looks like. I asked Dave if he thought they rigged the mirror to make people look thinner than they actually are. He walked over to the mirror wearing just his shorts, sort of frowned and said, "Nope!"

Wishing all of you peace and happiness as Spring arrives all around us.

Love,
Kathryn

UPDATE AT 8 MONTHS

Kathryn

April 9, 2015

It's truly Spring and a recent highlight for me was receiving a letter from the donor of my Jersey cells. A year ago right now I had gotten word from the Search department that finding a donor for me would be difficult, and maybe not possible. I spent a lot of time thinking about dying, and also about what a burden my illness would be for my family and friends. I also thought about what the experience would teach me about life and living, whether a donor could be found or not. Having found a donor, I now have a better than 50-50 chance of being alive in 7 years, which would not have been true without one. Once I learned that a donor had been found I was allowed to send her an anonymous thank you through her blood center. No other donor/ recipient contact is permitted until a year after the transplant. I can imagine possible reasons for that restriction and I was told that sometimes recipients have actually blamed donors for post-transplant problems--hard to imagine feeling anything but gratitude toward donors. I do know that my donor is a 33-year-old woman who is married with 2 kids and she lives somewhere in New Jersey. I expect we will both want to be in touch when a year has passed and I would hope to meet her someday.

The most exciting news at our house is that I got my Hickman central line out last Friday. It feels like a milestone and will be one less chore for Dave. We used the line for many home IV infusions and it required flushing before and after each use. Dave calculated quite a while ago that he had done these flushes over 2,000 times and he also had to do my dressing changes each week. He has been a reliable and good-humored caregiver during all of this but I'm enthused about being pretty self-reliant at this point. For over 30 years, my number one stress reduction strategy has been taking a hot bath with a good book and a shot of whiskey at night. I haven't been able to have a bath since July 18th but plan to have one tomorrow night to celebrate (!) I also got rid of the heart monitor and nothing ominous was found. I was told that I may have atrial fibrillation again at some point but I'm not planning on it.

I have been shifting my perspective on prednisone in ways that I hope will serve me well. I have been most worried about the long-term effects on bone density and joints, not so much about all the immediate side effects. I have been aware of taking the words of providers to heart. Having a doctor say, "If you're off all of your immune suppression at 6 months..." made me think that was a real possibility. Being told that my first prednisone taper would end November 20th of last year made me think I would be off it then and might escape long-term problems from the drug, even though I did know there was a chance I'd have to go on it again at some point. Having those kinds of hopes has led me to feeling like a central part of my recovery is "waiting" to get off prednisone. I have written about "waiting" before. I am still in the lab a lot and always think of people around the world anxiously waiting for news of all kinds--related to health, accidents, missing loved ones. A lot of waiting is inevitable on this path but it's a feeling that can lead to useless anxiety and a sense of living for some future day. Since I am 8 months into recovery and still on high dose prednisone, I have come to realize that there is no end of it in sight and I may be on it for years. I need to stay out of the "waiting" frame of mind, focus on the present, and do all I can to minimize short and long term side effects.

Immunoglobulins help protect us from infections and mine are lower than they should be at this point. I spent a morning this week getting an infusion of immunoglobulins from someone else to help reduce my risk of infections. Even though I am vulnerable to infections and have some physical problems, I am always surprised when someone refers to me being "sick." For some reason, during all of this I haven't thought of myself as someone with health problems; physically challenged for sure but not sick. I can't say I think of myself as "healthy" just yet but I do hope that day will come.

As I begin to re-engage with the world, I am really lucky that I am not under pressure to get back to paid work. I am exploring options for volunteering that don't involve being around people much, like maybe peer support by phone for transplant patients. My work has always been people packed, and I miss that, but I am still being cautious about exposing myself to crowds.

I am also working on getting our old house ready to sell next year since we haven't given up the idea of moving back to Vashon. There isn't much medical infrastructure there but there are lots of compassionate volunteers of all kinds. I have days when I feel like I have no business living someplace where a Fire Department volunteer with limited training might show up to handle a medical emergency if I called 911. Even so, I am not inclined to live my life next to an Urgent Care just in case I need one. We hope to start building this summer and get the shell up. We can then chip away at the inside work over the winter and move next year.

As we begin to see a pinhole view of a future that doesn't revolve around my health issues, I find myself looking back over this past year. I am so grateful to all of you for your love and support and good humor. Knowing we have friends and family on our strong team has made all the difference to us getting through the challenges.

With heartfelt thanks and good wishes to you in spring,

Kathryn

FAREWELL TO FLUSHES AND ALIEN SPACESHIPS

Dave

April 19, 2015

Day +267: Kathryn has shared the momentous news that her Hickman Central IV line was removed about 2 weeks ago after being in place for about 9 months. This feels like a huge milestone for both of us, and means that we are not quite so tethered together every single day. It also means that we can go away for the weekend without taking an extra suitcase filled with infusion bags, syringes, tubing, heparin and saline flushes, alcohol swabs, plastic gloves, and a few other pieces of essential equipment. Although this is obviously a great relief and a big step forward towards a more normal way of life, I must say that a small part of me will be wistful and will feel a sense of loss. Our daily routine of washing, gloving up, and carefully swabbing the claves on the end of the Y-shaped tubes coming out of Kathryn's chest and attending to their needs was a very intimate and loving ritual during some dark days, weeks and months. For the math geeks among you I can now give you the final tally during this time:

- **39 dressing changes**
- **593 infusions (mostly of magnesium but with a few "hand-grenades" of gancyclovir thrown in)**
- **1,232 heparin flushes**
- **1,837 saline flushes**
- **3,807 alcohol swabs**

As we both take deep breaths and take stock of where we are now and what still lies ahead I am reminded of two very dark periods in the past 12 months that are now behind us.

A year ago right now we still didn't know if there was any hope for Kathryn as a suitable donor had not yet been found and she was needing blood transfusions every few weeks to keep her blood counts up since her own bone marrow was rapidly failing, her energy level was slipping, and her spirit was faltering. We were having very different conversations with each other during those spring evenings than we are this April.

A couple of months ago was actually another really dark time for us. Kathryn still needed magnesium infusions every day. She had just been switched from tacrolimus to sirolimus to try to improve the situation and to see if that would work better along with the prednisone to keep her liver function tests staying down. She had had a second episode of funny fast heart rhythm (Atrial Fibrillation) and so the cardiologist wanted her to wear a continuous heart monitor 24 hours a day for a month to see what that showed. Her hip and back were hurting more and more so Kathryn couldn't do her routine of walking round the park and climbing 1000 stairs every day which not only helped keep her muscles and bones in better shape but helped with her mental health too. The doctors at Seattle Cancer Care Alliance said they thought that this hip pain might well mean that she was developing avascular necrosis of the hip bone (a condition where the ball at the upper end of the long thigh bone crumbles and dies because it can't get enough blood supply to it). This is one of the dreaded complications of high dose prednisone therapy in people after stem cell transplantation because it either results in you spending the rest of your life limping and in a state of chronic pain or hoping that you are fit enough to undergo hip replacement surgery on top of everything else that you are dealing with.

So our nights in bed together during those days were another kind of intimate experience altogether. Kathryn not only had her Hickman line tubes coming out of her chest and tucked into a small cloth bag attached to a lanyard around her neck she also had a rolled up bath towel tied around her waist like a python, to try to make her hip and back pain less uncomfortable during the night. Besides all of that she had three electrodes stuck onto her chest attached by wires to a recoding device (about the size of a cell phone) and a transmitting device (also about the size of a cell phone) clipped to the waistband of her pajamas. Both these devices flashed green, blue and red lights and emitted beeps from time to time. So our romantic nights in bed would be punctuated by incidents like this. It is 3am and I am drifting in and out of a light sleep trying to rest up for the day ahead. It is pitch dark and soothingly quiet. I roll over gently to try to put my arm around Kathryn and find some small piece of her that feels soft and warm and normal so that I can comfort her with a hug and a squeeze. Suddenly Kathryn flaps the covers off of both of us in her sleep because she is too hot. The room is instantly filled with green, blue and red lights flashing off the ceiling and beeping at me as if a 747 (or perhaps an alien spaceship) is coming in to land in the middle of the bedroom floor. The night is no longer soothingly quiet, the romance of the moment has evaporated, and I am rudely reminded of all the things that seem to be going wrong and that we still might have to face.

Compared with all of that, things really do seem to be moving forward in a more positive direction right now. We still have a long way to go and there are many other "bumps" large and small that we still have to avoid or deal with but we are both more than ready to move on and hope for some better days ahead and to start planning a future that contains more travel and adventure and fewer alcohol swabs and saline flushes... even though a small part of me will miss those days and look back on them with fondness for how much they kept Kathryn and me close. Still, I can think of quite a few other things that we could do together in the future that will keep us just as close and will be a LOT more fun.

KC'S PERSONAL LANDFILL

Dave: May 22, 2015

Day +300: This has been a landmark week for Kathryn and me in several ways. The fact that Kathryn is now officially 300 days post-stem cell transplant is a kind of artificial milestone but certainly means something to us. Probably the biggest sign that we are entering a new era was when I chatted to Kathryn today about other things and then, as an afterthought said,

"Oh, I forgot, how were your lab results this week?"

Kathryn continues to get her labs done every week but the fact that two days had gone by and I hadn't remembered to ask her what the results were is quite telling. For the past 6-7 weeks, now, they have been stable. I can't say that they are **normal** yet. It isn't normal to get a sirolimus level every week, or to hear that your cytomegalovirus (CMV) counts are undetectable. Her immunoglobulin levels are still too low and her liver function tests are staying at about twice the upper limit of normal but at least they are **stable.** We haven't had any unusual surprises now for several weeks, so I can almost forget to ask about the labs. Kathryn looks great and is functioning at about her usual pace and energy level again (which risks taking the paint off the walls as she "walks" through the house like the benevolent tornado that she is... a woman on a mission!).

We decided to start taking our accumulated transplant-related trash off to the dump. For the past 9 months we have gotten deliveries from Coram at least twice a week bringing us central line tubing, bags of fluids, saline and heparin syringes, alcohol swabs, batteries for the pump, etc, etc.) Every package came in a cardboard box lined with polystyrene foam with the syringes and infusion bags surrounded with frozen gel packs. There was way too much waste to go into our regular weekly Seattle garbage pick up and so we have been storing it in the shed under our deck in large plastic bags and boxes. This was enough to fill the back of my pickup truck several times over. Kathryn, who has always cared about the environment and who tries to leave a small footprint on the land has been embarrassed and unhappy at the amount of garbage that has been accumulating because of her. She has remarked more than once that she is creating a personal landfill all by herself and there were some dark days when she remarked that it might be better for everyone concerned and for the planet if I just took her and threw **her** into a landfill instead...

Needless to say we gave this option serious consideration (;-). It would certainly have made life simpler in some ways and might have given me some great plot ideas for a new murder mystery story... but on balance I decided that it would be better to keep Kathryn around and just throw away the trash that was accumulated in service of her recovery!

Neither of us has any illusions about being "out of the woods" just yet. Kathryn will have her 12-month evaluation at SCCA starting in early July. They will recheck her bone marrow and do a whole bunch of other tests. If she "passes" those tests they will give her all her childhood immunizations again. Until her new immune system is completely functional we need to keep reminding ourselves that right now Kathryn has the immunity of a newborn baby - she could get polio, measles, chicken pox, whooping cough, among other cosmic delights, anytime we let our guard down. She will remain immunosuppressed to some extent for at least another couple of years. We still need to be hyper vigilant about bleaching our cutting boards and washing every carrot stick and lettuce leaf in cold running water before drying it and putting it on a plate for Kathryn to eat. It still takes Kathryn hours and hours every day to go through her medical routines of careful bathing, applying creams and lotions, mouthwashes and rinses, counting pills and choking handfuls of them down with glasses of distilled water. And we are cursed with too much medical knowledge about all the possible complications and problems that **could** still be in our future.

But for the first time in about 18 months we can both begin to actually contemplate a future... a future that does not revolve around clinic and lab appointments or the constant 24-hours-a-day attention to every one of Kathryn's bodily functions. The fog is lifting just a little bit and we can catch glimpses of a different future... one where Kathryn is walking across fields of meadow grass on Vashon watching a pair of pileated woodpeckers quarreling in the apple trees... strolling down city streets in foreign countries chatting to street vendors or eating tapas at outside cafe tables late into a sultry summer evening... sitting by the log fire reading bedtime stories to grandkids sitting on her lap... standing on an empty beach on a remote Scottish island leaning into the wind... playing the piano in a new living room while her grand daughter plays along on the guitar... hiking along a snowy ridge in the Cascade mountains with friends...

Kathryn has enough energy, determination and imagination to dream up even more future adventures than those. I am just eternally grateful that she put herself through these many past grueling months to bring us to this point where all of that might just be possible. And although I know that I am just a little bit biased when I say this - in the grand scheme of things the amount of additional waste that Kathryn Crawford has added to the world's landfills is more than offset by the amount of joy, happiness, wisdom and support that she brings to everyone she meets.

GOOD NEWS AT ONE YEAR

Kathryn

July 12, 2015

Last week I had my series of annual exams and Dave and I were very happy to learn that there is no longer any sign of myelofibrosis in my body. My Jersey cells are producing red cells, white cells, and platelets in just the way we hoped they would. We have no way of knowing what kind of medical problems or complications might come up in the months or years ahead but in a way, that's true for all of us. Because of my ongoing graft-versus-host-disease, I will need to be on immune suppression medication for at least another year or two. Even so, I am lucky that my energy level seems about back to normal. I was hoping for three things at one year and I was told that swimming in Puget Sound, bouquets in the house, and even having a dog would be OK. Yahoo! My body has changed but otherwise I feel just like myself.

Dave and I feel lucky indeed to be going ahead with our plans to build a house on Vashon. Those plans have been on hold for a long time since a year ago we didn't know whether or not I would still be alive or fit for a project this big. We are getting our old house ready to sell, which is no small task, and will be moving to our family cabin in three weeks.

I suppose it's natural that, as the anniversary of my transplant arrives, every day we find ourselves thinking back to what we were doing a year ago. I was in the midst of two weeks of physical exams in preparation for my July 18th admission date. I had decided to go for it and it felt like I just needed to keep my eyes open, look straight ahead, and walk into the fire. Dave was preparing to be my official caregiver for 100 days. We knew the price of treatment would be high, financially and otherwise, and that there was no way of knowing anything about what the outcome might be. It feels like a milestone to have survived it thus far and feel well enough to be taking on moving and building again. Since we built a house before we know that moving and building are hard work, but these are total pleasure compared to what we were doing a year ago.

I really don't think I could have gotten through all this without Dave by my side. He has been with me every step of the way, from the somber weeks after my diagnosis last year to the toast we had to my health after my exams last week. He has been selfless, encouraging, energetic, and good-humored. I want to thank my wonderful family for acknowledging that the decision about whether or not to get a transplant was mine even though they were hoping I would get one. They have also supported me during all the ups and downs over the past year.

All the support we have received through Caring Bridge has also played a role in my healing and reminded me of what makes life worth living. As useful as Caring Bridge has been for us, the year milestone seems like a good time to stop posting updates and sign off. Since it turned out that neither Dave nor I had time to write journals of our own, our entries and the comments of love and encouragement will be a treasured record of this difficult year. I want to thank you for your emails, cards, phone calls, and offers of help of all kinds. Dave will want to write a closing entry of his own in the next few days. He also promised a post-transplant party some months ago and we will plan on that once we are moved into our new place, most likely next summer.

With wholehearted thanks and best wishes to all of you,

Kathryn

NO WALK IN THE PARK

Dave

July 14, 2015

Day +353: Last week came and went rather quietly. I wouldn't call it an anticlimax, but it was definitely uneventful... at least by the new standards that Kathryn and I have.

On Monday Kathryn went to the lab at SCCA where they drew eighteen tubes of blood. That's right... EIGHTEEN. But that was at least partly Kathryn's fault. She signed up for several research studies when all of this got going last year and all of those studies now require their "pound of flesh"... or at least their tubes of blood.

On Tuesday she had yet another bone marrow biopsy and so spent the rest of the day throwing up and feeling dizzy because of the "conscious sedation" they gave her that included a "Fentanyl Lollipop." But we were expecting that. No biggie.

On Wednesday Kathryn got her pulmonary function tests done again to see if GVHD was quietly destroying her lungs. Getting lung function tests involves breathing into tubes as fast and as hard as you can while some zealous technician yells, "Breathe harder... HARDER! DON'T STOP!" Nothing unusual there. Kathryn has done that before. After that a medical student asked Kathryn to walk laps along a corridor as fast as she could while she was being timed. At the end of that the student announced breathlessly that Kathryn had just completed more than twice as many laps as anyone she had ever tested before. I, for one, was not surprised by that statement.

Later that day Kathryn got a first dose of every one of her entire childhood immunizations since her previous lifelong immunity had been wiped out last July leaving her with less protection than a newborn. They made a map of all the suitable areas on Kathryn's body where they could happily stick their needles and squirt foreign substances under her skin. It was a reminder that for the past twelve months Kathryn has been totally vulnerable and could have gotten pneumonia, Hepatitis A or B, meningitis, whooping cough, diphtheria, tetanus, or polio if she had stumbled across any of those nasty little bugs. No worries, though. Just water under the bridge at this stage. We just need to remember to schedule all her booster shots over the next several months.

So on Thursday we sat down in a conference room with the head of the Long Term Follow-up Unit at SCCA - the incomparable Dr. Mary Flowers (accompanied by her usual entourage of fellows and physicians from France, Canada, Brazil...). Dr. Flowers went through

Kathryn's results with brisk efficiency.

"The news is all good. You have no fibrosis in your bone marrow. None. Is all gone. No signs of relapse. Relapse is possible, of course, but unlikely. Your lungs are good. Your blood counts are all normal. Your liver tests are stable. Your immunoglobulins are still low but we expect that at this stage. Getting all those immunizations will help the immunoglobulins increase faster.

You still have chronic GVHD, of course, but this is stable on low dose prednisone. I want to keep you on that along with the sirolimus for at least one more year, maybe more. The repeat dexa is stable. Is all good. So how are you feeling? What questions do you have?"

During all this time Kathryn had been looking over the two pages of neatly typed questions that she had prepared ahead of this meeting. She put check marks against all of the questions that had already been answered as Dr. Flowers had been talking. When Dr. Flowers asked her question Kathryn quickly scanned the list while about a dozen international eyes looked at her from around the conference table. As you can imagine Kathryn is rather shy and deferential in situations like this... she'll be stuck for words or might only ask vague, indirect, tentative questions, right?

"Thanks, I have one question to start with. With what you know about me right now and all the information you that you have gathered, what are the chances that GVHD will kill me in the next five years?"

That's my gal! Call it like you see it!

Dr. Flowers remained unfazed and straightforward. She checked the chart and rattled off a list of risk factors... How early the GVHD had started in

Kathryn's case, the presence or lack of thrombocytopenia at the onset of GVHD, the fact that high dose steroids had been needed during the first hundred days but were not needed now, and so forth...

"You strong... and fit... doing well. The chances of survival at five years for you? I'd say 85%. I'd like to see you again in six months."

So that was it. The entourage left and we moved on to the pharmacy consult to go over the pills and potions that Kathryn has to take at this stage. Now for a girl who used to take one single pill plus a multivitamin before all of this started the list may seem long, but compared to what we have been handling and dealing with in recent months the current med list is a "piece of cake."

- Prednisone 10mg every other day
- Sirolimus 1mg once a day
- Bactrim DS one pill every day
- Acyclovir 800mg twice a day
- Ursadiol 300mg twice a day
- Metoprolol 25mg once a day
- Raloxifine 60mg once a day
- Pravastatin 10mg once a day in the evening
- Vitamin D 1000mg every day
- Calcium citrate 1200mg every day
- Multivitamin once a day
- Dexamethasone 0.1mg per ml, rinse for four minutes 4 times a day
- Clotrimazole troches 10mg, 4 times every day
- Restasis 1 drop in each eye twice a day

- Fluoromethalone 0.1%, one drop in each eye 4 times every day
- Refresh eye drops hourly
- Estring every 3 months
- Sodium fluoride gel daily at bedtime

So here we are on **Day +353**. As I reflect back on these past eighteen months or so here are a few random things that I'd like to share with you.

I have maybe written more than I should have. I have certainly written more than Kathryn has and that's a shame because she always has great insights and wise things to share. Kathryn processes a lot more by talking to other people. I don't. I'm a writer. It helps me organize my thoughts and figure out how I feel if I write things down and try to explain them to other people.

I can't thank you all enough for the love and support that you have shown to me and to Kathryn during this difficult time. You have helped us in your own unique and different ways. We have especially appreciated the shared humor. This journey would have been much less bearable without all your support.

Having said that, I have never felt more lonely, ragged, and exposed at any time in my life as I have during these past eighteen months. That is not a reflection on any of you but is just what it has felt like to be living the hour-by-hour, day-by-day monotony and seeing the hellish misery that the love of my life has been going through.

We had some very pleasant surprises in amongst the misery and hard stuff, though...

We had a rare visit from Connie H, breezing in from Ecuador on her way to Nigeria like an exotic whiff of wacky wit and good humor. Connie is a great reminder of how many adventures are out there waiting for us in the big wide world.

Julie G has been a warm, deep, substantial presence throughout. Julie is wise and authentic, bold and direct. She was always interested in how we were really feeling. Whether she was off doing workshops in the Middle East or was holed up on Orcas, I always felt that her support was nearby at all times.

Gabriella M has tended to our garden with love and care during these past two seasons when neither of us was able to. Kathryn was forbidden to be burrowing around in soil up to her elbows the way she loves to do, in case she disturbed fungus spores into the air that might find their way to her lungs. And I wasn't too much help, either. I didn't feel that I had a waking second or a scintilla of energy left to devote to garden chores once all Kathryn's other essential needs were attended to. Yet our garden has never looked more exuberant and full of color, life and promise. It is hard to quantify the emotional and spiritual boost that that gave to Kathryn, but I know that it was, and still is, an important part of her recovery.

Tina S traveled across the country to visit us during some of our darkest days. She brought a delightful, quirky, thoughtful attitude and gave us some great perspective and conversation. She also brought us a Lyle Lovett CD ("Step Inside This House") and said, "You guys should listen to Track 8 on Disc 2. It always makes me think of you."

So Kathryn and I held onto each other as we listened to ***"If I Needed You"*** in the kitchen that night... and on many occasions since then. There is usually a pool of tears on the floor by the time the track is over. I'm pretty sure that those tears are just coming from Kathryn, though, and not from me. At least you can't tell whose they are if I am quick enough to wipe my face and the floor with a towel as soon as the song is done...

Our kids and extended family have been rock solid throughout all of this. They are a huge part of the reason why Kathryn has put herself through all of this.

I have a new, deep, and sincere appreciation for hand-sanitizer, bleach, and triple-washed lettuce leaves... and for how amazing a healthy immune system is!

If this had to happen at all I am grateful that this illness happened to Kathryn in **this** city and at **this** moment in history. Seattle is one of a very few true centers of excellence in the world for this field of medical research. If this had happened in the 1970s in Edinburgh where I was training at the time there would have been no hope of cure. No doubt in fifty more years people will look back and roll their eyes at how primitive and unenlightened the treatment for myelofibrosis was in 2014 but Kathryn and I know that what she has received is the absolute best treatment that is available right now and that her current and future life owes a lot to that.

Let me leave you with a few final thoughts as we close our Caring Bridge journal. We hope to see many of you in person as the months and years go on, and, as Kathryn mentioned, we will have a celebratory party at our new house on Vashon once that has been built and we have moved in next year.

Yesterday afternoon Kathryn and I walked (briskly, of course!) around the Discovery Park Loop Trail for about the thousandth time. We reflected on how this walk has felt to us at different stages on our Uncertain Journey.

In the spring of last year, before Kathryn got admitted to the transplant unit, at a time when her blood counts kept dropping rapidly, and repeatedly we could gauge how well she was doing by how breathless she got and how fast her pulse raced as we walked along the trail. If I could keep up with her easily and she was panting then her hematocrit was probably below 25 and she needed to get another blood transfusion.

In August, just after Kathryn got discharged from the transplant unit we walked round the loop trail with some trepidation as she got magnesium or Micofungin delivered directly through a vein into the base of her heart from the infusion pump in her back pack... the one that sounded like Darth Vader.

Later in the year we had to cover the infusion pump and back pack in plastic bags and cinch them up tight with twist ties so that we could get our miles in while the cold Pacific Northwest rain thundered down through the leafy canopy above our heads. We smelled the loamy mulch of fallen leaves decaying in the fall. We felt the crunch of frost under our feet over the winter. We rejoiced in the Fifty Shades of Green that erupted from the ground and the branches this past spring. And here we are again in the dusty heat of summer... still walking briskly around the loop, but at a very different point in our lives.

After going through what we have been through (and I know we are not done yet!) I am not sure what advice I would now give to an anxious stranger contemplating whether or not to sign up for a stem cell transplant. I can't decide what suggestions I might offer to their caregiver. How well a person does depends on so many factors, both known and unknown. There is no way to know how successful any person's treatment will be. It depends a lot on what the particular underlying disease is that has necessitated the stem cell transplant. It depends in part on the immunological subtleties in the match from a stranger's hematopoietic stem cells. It depends, in part, on how each person defines success. For me, personally, no matter how things go from this point forward I am eternally grateful that Kathryn put herself through all of this. I didn't "need" this in my life to see what a remarkable human being Kathryn is. I knew that already. I didn't "need" to be put through this to test the depth of my own character. I wouldn't wish this on anyone and yet I know that many thousands of people around the world will go through their own version of this. Their own Uncertain Journey. I have no specific words of advice, no particular wise or comforting insights except maybe to mention a few things that I have learned from Kathryn along the way. This is an incomplete list of what makes up "The Kathronian Way."

Stay real. Be present in all the moments, good and bad. Stay curious and open to learning. Be humble, but be confident in yourself. If you need to make a big decision try to find at least three options, write down the pros and cons of each option... and then make a decision and don't look back. Share how you really feel with those you feel close to. Find humor wherever you can. Give comfort and courage to others. Whenever possible stay patient and optimistic, but when you feel impatient, angry and despondent... let it rip! Set aside time to have a good blubber whenever you think it might

help.

In all the things I have written over this past year and a half I have used plenty of tortured metaphors! But I have studiously tried to avoid using sporting or warfare metaphors. To me those are tired and overused in cancer narratives. I have not been able to avoid metaphors involving journeys, though. I have taken you over metaphorical mountains, down into the Pit of Despair, and along many winding highways and byways with bumps in the road and potholes along the way. So let me leave you with one more. While there are many things I might say to a stranger contemplating going ahead with a stem cell transplant there is one thing that I would **not** say. Despite all the references that Kathryn and I have made to the restorative part that our walks along the Discovery Park Loop Trail have played in our recovery, I would never tell anyone that what we are going through is an easy path to take. There are many ways to describe what is involved with getting a bone marrow/stem cell transplant. But one thing is certain.

It is **No Walk In The Park.**

FIVE YEARS ON

Dave

March 2nd, 2019

Day +1,679: Okay, I confess that we are not still tracking things in terms of how many days Kathryn is post transplant, but if we were today would be Day +1,679. In a few months she will pass the five-year mark. Dr. Mary flowers told Kathryn in July 2015 at her one-year evaluation that she thought Kathryn had an 85% chance of being alive at five years. It looks like we are going to make that milestone. I know that if Kathryn had not put herself through this she would have died three or four years ago. So my main reflection at this point is immense gratitude to the team who helped get Kathryn to this point and to Kathryn for the undaunted courage she has shown throughout all of this. Incidentally, ***Undaunted Courage: Meriwether Lewis, Thomas Jefferson, and the Opening of the American West, by Stephen E. Ambrose*** is one of Kathryn's favorite books. She had read it more than once long before she and I embarked on our own uncertain journey.

Since my last Caring Bridge entry, four years ago, things have not really "settled down." We never feel we can totally relax or take Kathryn's "stable bad" health for granted. Her graft-versus-host-disease (GVHD) continues to attack her body in a variety of ways. Some of these have been merely annoying, others have been life-threatening. I marvel that she spends half of all her waking hours dealing with chores just to maintain the quality of life that she has. She still has to track massive numbers of drugs: twenty-three different pills or potions to swallow, inhale, or slather on various body parts. She has to ensure that she doesn't run out of anything if we are out of town visiting family or friends. She sets alarms on her phone to remind her to take particular drugs because some need to be taken with food, others on an empty stomach, yet others that can't be taken within an hour or two of other drugs. The brand, color, size and shape of the pills change from time to time. Avoiding pharmacological disaster requires Kathryn's constant attention. She carries eye drops with her at all times and has to lubricate her eyeballs every few minutes and take out, clean, and reinsert her massive scleral lenses several times a day. She does exercise of all sorts for a couple of hours every day, and still has more medical and laboratory appointments than most people our age.

Yet Kathryn virtually never complains. She jokes that she has a half-time job doing "body maintenance," and regrets that this keeps her from engaging with the rest of the world as much as she would like to. Even so, she manages to do lots of interesting things during the other half of her waking hours. She is involved in community events and we take great pleasure in events big and small in our family and around the world. I don't think that Kathryn or I ever took our lives or good health for granted. It shouldn't take a major traumatic event to make a person appreciate the precious life that we have. But there is no doubt that going through this with Kathryn has changed the way I look at things. While I wouldn't wish what we have gone through on anyone I truly appreciate the life experience that it has given me. I started this narrative with a statement of the obvious. "Life, itself, is an uncertain journey." I will end by saying how extremely happy and grateful that my journey through life with Kathryn Crawford is continuing.

Kathryn

At this point I have accepted that I will never be "out of the woods," and yet the transplant success was a miracle. My Jersey Girls had just gotten warmed up with the GVHD by the time we stopped Caring Bridge. It took some soul searching and adjusting expectations to accept that my life will never back to what my peers and I think of as "normal." I will always have some feeling of not being in the same world as my friends, who are doing things like bicycling in Cuba and backpacking in other countries. I love change and travel and novelty and all of those are challenging for me now. Even so, every now and then I am suddenly struck with a feeling of overwhelming gratitude, and astonishment really, that I am still here and able to do as much as I can. And I've learned my lesson about waiting for things to get better. I try to appreciate everything I can about each day the sunrise brings.

In some ways, the acute hospital part of the ordeal was the easy part. During periods of acute illness or hospitalization we feel we have "permission" to drop everything and focus on our health, and people gather round to support us. As we enter the long period of recovery we must try to resume some sort of "normal" lives and the supporters have to resume theirs. It has become clear that recovering from a transplant is a marathon, not a sprint. One of the things I miss most from my pre-transplant life is the relative complacency about my health. It now feels like I have a file on almost every body part. I did not take my health for granted before my transplant but health challenges were not front and center every day in the way they are now. I've had a hard time getting the hang of identifying myself as "vulnerable." I am at risk for various things that I need to be vigilant about avoiding, such as infections, skin injuries from prednisone, broken bones from falls, sun exposure, and a variety of other things. I still have to be very careful about what I eat whether I am at home or out. I vacillate now between thinking I should be extra careful about food additives and pesticides to thinking I'm so polluted already that maybe it doesn't really make any difference. Being instructed to be careful about all kinds of things doesn't feel normal to me because I have always felt robust. I have been very lucky to rarely have even gotten colds but when I get "sick," I do it in a big way.

I am a public health nurse and I have loved my public health work. I had planned to return to work of some kind after my transplant but it became clear that that was not a realistic hope. That was a big loss but I was incredibly lucky to be able to consider myself retired since Dave was employed. I have always been focused on meaning in my work and I recognized that I would have to find meaningful activities beyond my family.

One of the things that was most striking to me throughout my experience was how very rarely I was ever asked how I was doing as a whole person, not simply how I would assess some particular symptom. As a nurse, I believed one of the most important things for me to know about a patient was how they were doing as a person, not simply as a patient. I didn't want to appear ungrateful to my wonderful providers but I wanted them to more often acknowledge the burden of living with my symptoms, as well as living with the major uncertainty about the quality of my life in the future.

I think more thought should be given to how expectations are set prior to major treatments as serious as transplants. It will be tough for providers of all kinds to gauge what the best way to do this is for each patient. Even so, they would have some clues if patients were asked things such as, "What's most important to you as you consider this treatment? What are you most worried about? What do you hope for most as a result of the treatment?" It seems important to bear in mind that it is no kinder to set expectations that are overly optimistic than it is to undermine hopes. I have imagined that for many people creating a qualified hope such as, "You may be able to backpack but you shouldn't count on it" might set the right tone. I have always had a lot of energy and I am an adventuresome person. I have many more limits than I anticipated even though I recognized that there was no way to know ahead of time how things might go. I do think expectations for how I would do were set too high but I also recognize that I may have heard what I wanted to to some degree.

I have had many serious and fairly uncommon

problems since we closed our Caring Bridge account in the summer of 2015. I have tried hard to befriend my Jersey Girls from the beginning, talking to them, bribing them. It seems like such a paradox that they are making perfectly healthy blood for me but also wreaking havoc with much of my body. My hair never came back and on good days one of my doctors refers to my eye problems as "stable bad." I have atrial fibrillation, my lung function is compromised, and I have sclerosis in my feet and legs. Half my fingernails and all my toenails are deformed and starting to come off. Don't take your fingernails for granted, it's quite a functional impairment not having them. Since the summer of 2015 I have been on more drugs and clinical trial drugs, and I did nine months of extracorporeal photopheresis. In 2017 I developed nephrotic syndrome and it was unclear for about a month whether or not I would survive. That meant being back on crazy making doses of prednisone for months. (Transplant doses of prednisone are high (50 mg/day for me) and the dose is tapered down very slowly with hopes that my GVHD doesn't flare up. I still have the champagne we were going to drink when I got off my first prednisone taper on November 20th of 2014. I'm still on it. Some of the common side effects of prednisone include insomnia, moodiness, anxiety, loss of muscle and bone, irritability, weight gain, and trouble thinking. I didn't understand ahead of time how up and down the prednisone doses would be. A transplant nurse told me that they hope to provide people with "a little taste of life that they would not otherwise have had." In spite of all my problems, I feel like I have actually had a big bite of life since my transplant. I have backpacked with friends, traveled close to home, had wonderful times with kids, and Dave and I have built a new house.

I am asked often how I manage to keep going. For thirty years my primary stress management strategy was a very hot bath each night with a book and a shot of whiskey. I gave that up for a couple of years due to sclerosis activation in my feet. I am thrilled that my foot problems have calmed down and I'm back to bathing. I do have a lot of problems but also a lot of good fortune. I can eat well and continue to exercise in the way that I have for my whole life. I have a wonderful place to live and a garden that feeds my soul. I have the support of family and friends, and the love and support of my husband, Dave. I find it hard to believe but he assures me that he is thankful that I went through with the transplant and he wouldn't want to be anywhere else. He's a gem.

For some reason I have always been pretty aware of my mortality and have been deliberate about keeping my actions lined up with my values. Even so, I am more aware of my mortality now in a day to day way. I take extra pleasure in seeing the moon over our meadow, hearing frogs in the spring, having coffee with a friend. I make no assumptions about how long I will live or, for that matter, how long people I love will live. I have what I describe as a tiny meditation practice that I have had for many years. I believe the grounding it provides has been a key part of why I have often been told during these years that I just seem like myself. I once read about an old city motto in Paris that I feel like I could take as my own. **Fluctuat nec mergitur.** Translated from Latin it is:

Tossed but not sunk.

Kathryn Leigh Crawford grew up in the Pacific Northwest and has always loved the outdoors. She is an avid gardener and hiker. Her work as a Public Health nurse has focused on people with limited resources. She and Dave met in 1986 and they have been together ever since.

David Kennedy McCulloch grew up in a quiet rural backwater of Scotland where his dad was the village schoolteacher. He works as a doctor in the Pacific Northwest and is the author of the Wullie-The-Mahaar-Gome fantasy fiction series (www.tiny.cc/wulliesworld).

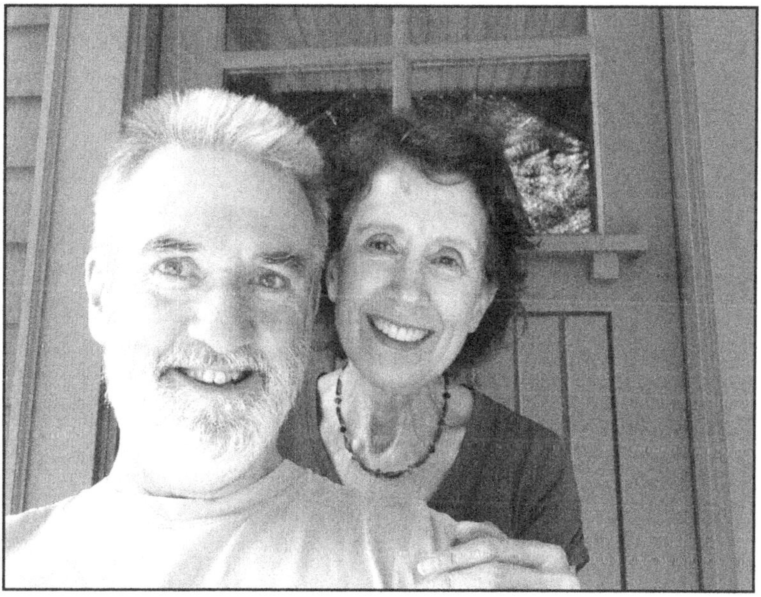

An Uncertain Journey is also available as an ebook and audiobook. Learn more and chat with Kathryn and Dave at:

http://www.tiny.cc/uncertainjourney

Made in the USA
Monee, IL
04 November 2026

67387463R10184